Advance Praise
Physician Well-Being

"Yellowlees builds on his seminal work on physician suicide with another brilliant series of illustrative narratives that lay out the root causes, and solutions, of the crisis in physician burnout, depression, and suicide. This is. . . by far the most comprehensive and readable work I have seen on this subject. Everything from underlying personality factors in physicians to medical marriages, financial literacy, and systemic factors such as implicit bias, loss of autonomy, and electronic medical records is covered. . . to lay out what's happening in contemporary medicine in the United States. This book brings a beacon of hope to those medical students, residents, and attending physicians working in an ailing system of care and has never been more needed than right now."

Steven Wengel, M.D., Professor of Psychiatry, Assistant Vice Chancellor for Campus Wellness, University of Nebraska Medical Center

"Dr. Yellowlees has come through once again. His skill in storytelling serves to illustrate concrete solutions to the current crisis of physician wellness and burnout."

Rajiv Misquitta, M.D., FACP, past President, Sierra Sacramento Valley Medical Society (SSVMS), and Chair, SSVMS Joy of Medicine committee

"Yellowlees. . . has prepared an engaging and comprehensive guide to the issues and solutions involved with physician wellness. This is a wonderful follow up to his first book [*Physician Suicide: Cases and Commentaries*]. . . . These two books are the first I have encountered to truly address the multifaceted issues in physician wellness and can jointly be used as textbooks in the field."

Anju Hurria M.D., M.P.H., Associate Clinical Professor, Department of Psychiatry, and Director of Medical School and Faculty Wellness Program, University of California Irvine

"This book takes a novel approach to presenting and reviewing material related to physician well-being. . . . For the reader who seeks to understand the important nuances of physician health and well-being, this publication is a treasure trove of salient topics."

Karen Miotto, M.D.

Physician Well-Being

CASES AND SOLUTIONS

Physician Well-Being

CASES AND SOLUTIONS

Peter Yellowlees, MBBS, M.D.

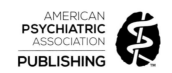

AMERICAN
PSYCHIATRIC
ASSOCIATION
PUBLISHING

First Edition

Manufactured in the United States of America on acid-free paper
24   23   22   21   20   5   4   3   2   1

American Psychiatric Association Publishing
800 Maine Avenue SW
Suite 900
Washington, DC 20024-2812
www.appi.org

Library of Congress Cataloging-in-Publication Data
Names: Yellowlees, Peter, author. | American Psychiatric Association, issuing body.
Title: Physician well-being : cases and solutions / Peter Yellowlees.
Description: First edition. | Washington, DC : American Psychiatric Association Publishing, [2020] | Includes bibliographical references and index.
Identifiers: LCCN 2019046650 (print) | LCCN 2019046651 (ebook) | ISBN 9781615372409 (paperback ; alk. paper) | ISBN 9781615372904 (ebook)
Subjects: MESH: Physicians—psychology | Burnout, Professional—prevention & control | Organizational Culture | Work-Life Balance | Education, Medical—organization & administration | Case Reports
Classification: LCC BF481 (print) | LCC BF481 (ebook) | NLM W 21 | DDC 158.7/ 23—dc23
LC record available at https://lccn.loc.gov/2019046650
LC ebook record available at https://lccn.loc.gov/2019046651

British Library Cataloguing in Publication Data
A CIP record is available from the British Library.

This book is dedicated to all the physicians whom I have treated as my patients over the past few decades in both Australia and the United States of America. They have taught me so much about the profession of medicine and what an honor it is to practice in this most meaningful occupation.

CONTENTS

About the Author ix

Preface xi

Acknowledgments xxi

Chapter 1

"Our Dedicated Dad" 1

Chapter 2

Health Care Is a Team Sport 27

Chapter 3

A Unified Mission 53

Chapter 4

Trust, Mentoring, and Innovation 77

Chapter 5

Pre-Med: Vulnerability and Trauma 101

Chapter 6

Medical School: Implicit Biases and
a Well-Being Curriculum 125

Chapter 7

Residency:
A Narcotic Addict's New Career 149

Chapter 8

Cognitive Dissonance and
Defining Meaning in Medicine 169

Chapter 9

Medical Marriages:
Caring for Each Other 193

Chapter 10

The Joy and Meaning of Medicine 215

Index 235

ABOUT THE AUTHOR

PETER YELLOWLEES, MBBS, M.D., is the Alan Stoudemire Endowed Professor of Psychiatry at University of California (UC) Davis in Sacramento, California. He is also Chief Wellness Officer for UC Davis Health and Vice Chair for Faculty Development in the Department of Psychiatry at UC Davis School of Medicine. He is a past President of the American Telemedicine Association. After completing his medical training in London, Dr. Yellowlees worked in Australia for 20 years, where he completed his research doctorate at Flinders University and became Chair of the Department of Psychiatry at the University of Queensland, before moving to UC Davis to continue his research in 2004. He has an international reputation in telemedicine and long-distance health and education delivery and has for many years treated physicians as patients. Dr. Yellowlees has worked in public and private sectors, in academia, and in rural settings. He has published 7 books and more than 200 scientific articles and book chapters and has been the author and video presenter of the internationally viewed "Medscape Psychiatry Minute" since 2009. He has been regularly involved in media presentations and has consulted to governments and private sector companies in several countries.

PREFACE

THIS IS MY SECOND BOOK on the topic of physician health. In my first book, *Physician Suicide: Cases and Commentaries*, published in 2018, I focused on the causes of distress and available treatments for physicians affected by it, mainly as individuals. I use the same style in this book; each chapter consists of a long, detailed case description of a component of physicians' lived experiences, followed by a commentary examining the major themes and referencing key works or papers from the literature. Yet this book is very different from the first. As the title suggests, in *Physician Well-Being: Cases and Solutions* I focus primarily on solutions that work to improve the health and well-being of physicians and other health care providers. These solutions are mainly systemic and organizational. They not only will reduce the high levels of suicide and burnout experienced by many physicians but also, equally importantly, will improve patient care and patient safety. If implemented widely, they will make our health care systems more effective as our populations age and medical practice continues to become more complicated. The two books can be read in sequence with relatively little overlap between them, but they each have a rather different philosophical approach. As a combination, they provide a comprehensive review of physician health and well-being and the professional and personal lifestyles of today's physicians.

It is important to begin with an agreed set of facts about physician health, as I have recently described (Yellowlees 2019), starting with our physical health. From a physical perspective, physicians look after themselves well and live on average 2 years longer than nonphysicians in the general population because, on the whole, we apply to ourselves the same advice we give our patients about the behavioral causes of medical illnesses. We tend not to smoke, to eat reasonably, and to exercise regularly. As a result, we tend not to be obese. Consequently, we generally have less chronic cardiovascular and respiratory illness than the general population, which leads to our relative longevity, despite the fact that we frequently treat ourselves and that many of us do not regularly see a primary care practitioner.

What about our mental health? How do physicians compare with the general population here? Not so well, unfortunately. Most medical students start medical school at ages 22–24 years, and we know that at that time they are more resilient and less depressed than equivalent graduate students in other disciplines. So, we start out well, having often overcome a number of childhood adverse events and proved our resiliency by jumping through the very high hoops associated with medical school entry. However, within a few years this changes, and numerous studies have documented increasing levels of burnout and depression during medical school and residency. It is now widely accepted that 10–15 years after entering medical school, the average physician has twice the level of burnout of the average professional nonphysician, primarily caused by systemic and organizational issues.

In terms of general mental health, physicians have all the same mental health problems as community control subjects except in relation to three areas:

1. Physicians tend to have a smaller prevalence of schizophrenia than the community, because symptom onset usually occurs prior to the age physicians enter medical school, although physicians' rates of bipolar disorder are similar.
2. Both male and female physicians exhibit the same, and higher, rates of death from suicide than the nonphysician community, in which males typically use more lethal means and therefore die from suicide more commonly than females. Female physicians die from suicide at twice the rate of community control subjects, whereas male physicians die from suicide at 1.4 times the rate. Rates of suicide are related to depression, often caused by chronic exposure to trauma on a daily basis, and here female physicians in particular exceed community rates.
3. Although physician rates of alcohol abuse disorder match those of the general community, physician abuse of prescribed drugs, such as narcotics and benzodiazepines, is more common than among community control groups, and their abuse of nonprescribed or illicit drugs, such as methamphetamine, heroin, and cocaine, is significantly less common.

I am passionate about the topic of physician well-being. After practicing as a psychiatrist for more than 30 years, and having treated many hundreds of physicians as patients, I believe that the health of physicians, the most important group of healers in our worldwide health systems, can no longer be ignored. If we buy a new car, it automatically comes with a long-term maintenance program for which we are happy to pay because we know that the car will last longer, and drive better and more safely, if we keep it well maintained. Similarly, but on the human side, anyone who wishes to become a professional athlete knows that they will need to take great care of both their body and their mind if they are to succeed at the highest level. They need to train and rest regularly, eat and sleep well, and have continuous coaching for both physical and psychological needs. They also need the support of trainers, family, friends, other athletes, and team members as well as fans in order to regularly perform at their best and at the highest level. When they have an injury or are not performing well, they need extra help and support and, possibly, time off to recover.

Both of these example metaphors apply perfectly to physicians, except we do not provide ourselves such maintenance and support programs anywhere near the degree to which we need them. This book is full of examples of how such programs can be introduced and maintained and how changes in the culture and process of medicine are both possible and essential.

At a personal level, I have been fortunate to live in four different countries during my life, and I have practiced medicine in three of them: England, Australia, and the United States. It has been evident to me for many years that doctors are of a similar quality in terms of their training, clinical capacities, and ethical perspectives in all three countries, yet the culture of the medical systems in which they work is very different, as are the pressures and stresses applied every day to physicians. Despite their cultural differences, the three countries are similar in one respect: None pays more than passing recognition to the importance of physician health, and none of them takes this issue seriously or is attempting to address it properly.

With this background, when as a psychiatrist I see physicians as patients, I always try to take account of the culture in which they trained and are working as well as the individual problems that have led to them being referred to me. After treating many physicians with all manner of psychiatric disorders, the one really obvious fact that I have learned is that physicians on the whole are very resilient and thoughtful patients, once they make the leap to become patients and stop trying to treat themselves or ignore their symptoms. At that stage, they almost always want to get well and will work hard to do so. They can learn to trust another physician and are generally very rewarding to treat. They all struggle working within the health care system, but they do their best to help their patients despite all the barriers put in their way.

In this book you will read about ways to overcome many of these barriers. It should become obvious that the major reasons for physician distress are organizational and systemic and that physicians are not themselves primarily to blame, except for their past lack of insight and unpreparedness to ask for help with their own health care. I hope that you will take a broad look at the major "elephants" in the room relating to physician health and well-being, including, in no particular order, the hours we are expected to work in the United States as residents and attending physicians; the current and worsening physician workforce shortages, especially in primary care and psychiatry; and the hours of administrative "busy work" (simple administrative tasks that could be done easily by others) we are required and expected to do. These hours, usually spent on a computer, are required to justify orders and prescriptions and to satisfy the demands of the electronic medical record (EMR) as well as the malignant health insurance industry, which is increasingly inserting itself into our daily work. Terms such as "pajama time" (time spent working on the EMR after hours) and "note bloat" (excess clinical documentation) have entered our lexicon. The spread of our work activities into our homes and social lives has made the concept of a "work-life balance" a distant hope for many. We all know that the practice of medicine has become more complicated, requiring more knowledge of novel tests and treatments and more specialization and involving more severe chronic illness and higher patient and community expectations—all to be delivered in the same length of consultation as 30 years ago. Combine these factors with the crushing graduate and medical school debt we accumulate, the inherent competitiveness of most medical disciplines, and our professional culture of denial, avoidance, and lack of self or collegial care—to name a few unintended adverse consequences of our professional code of ethics and behaviors—and it is hardly surprising that burnout and related conditions are rampant among physicians.

However, despite all this, I am optimistic about the future. We can reduce our "busy work," tame the EMR and finally make it useful, and change our professional culture. Many solutions are out there, and I look forward to sharing them with you. Some are potentially massive and will take generations to occur, such as philosophical and practical approaches to shortening the work week and beliefs about the need for holidays and time off. Others are technical and complicated, such as reducing the amount of documentation physicians put into the EMR, thereby creating better notes that require less need for working at midnight on a Sunday, or improving clinical workflows to keep all practitioners working at the top of their licenses. Other solutions are simple and attitudinal, such as learning how to confront problems rather than deny them or how to ask colleagues how they are feeling and then support them without judgment.

We still have a great deal to learn about physician well-being, and I hope that between us, we will gradually change the culture of medicine and reduce the numbers of physicians who become burned out or, even more tragically, die from suicide. We have far to go, but I hope this book is a positive step along the way. I have most certainly not covered all of the solutions, because they change constantly, and new initiatives and projects are being regularly described. I wanted to move away from the drama and distress that tend to arise whenever the latest high levels of, for example, burnout or suicide, are announced and instead describe case studies in which physicians and their colleagues from other disciplines succeed in overcoming the many forces working to keep them apart from their patients and loved ones. After all, I have never met a physician who told me that he or she went into medicine in order to spend 30% more of the working day on administrative requirements and clinical documentation. Yet that is what most now are doing, and it must stop. This book is an attempt at a clinical case–driven guide giving a series of examples of how this can be stopped and how the lives and lifestyles of physicians and other medical providers can be improved.

Before we look at the solutions, however, it is important to perform a scan of the U.S. health care industry. It is broadly known and understood that the United States has both the best and the worst of everything in health care. Magnificent systems of care, with specialty expertise at unparalleled levels, are demonstrated by Kaiser Permanente, the Mayo and Cleveland Clinic systems, and many academic systems such as Johns Hopkins, Harvard, and the University of California. Highly trained providers and world-class facilities are available in every state. However, large numbers of uninsured or underinsured patients are also still out there, as are bloated and overpaid health insurance and pharmaceutical industries that have been unable to help the thousands of Americans dying from opioid abuse and dependence each year. All this occurs in a health system that is not a system at all but that costs—at 18% of gross domestic product—more than any equivalent Western health system and delivers worse per-capita care than most Western countries.

This is a "health system"—a term I use generously—under major stress. In this system, physicians as a group are the first to really show this stress, as though they are a vulnerability marker for a system with a serious medical illness. Physicians are the equivalent of canaries in a coal mine. In medicine, in this situation, we typically try to diagnose what is going wrong before we decide on a course of treatment. This book is about the treatment, and the solutions, for physicians as a group, but the ultimate solution is broad improvement in the health system and organization. The causes of our impaired and sick health system are many and longstanding, but they are also beyond the scope of this book. The immediate stressors, however, are not. As the two major political parties continue to fight over the Affordable Care Act (ACA), leading to continuing uncertainty about the direction for U.S. health care over the next 10 years or so, a number of broad stressors are currently affecting American health care and are well worth mentioning to give context to the solutions offered here.

Darrell Kirch, M.D., is one of American medicine's most visionary leaders. For more than a decade he has been president and chief executive officer (CEO) of the Association of American Medical Colleges, which represents the nation's medical schools, teaching hospitals, and academic societies. He is one of the most thoughtful and creative leaders in American medicine and has given a number of talks focused on the likely disruptive changes that will affect the American medical community over the next decade. Although his main focus is on academic medical centers, with their three primary missions of clinical care, research, and education, his description of the upcoming profound disruptions to health care given to the American College of Psychiatrists in February 2019 is relevant to all sectors, and particularly with respect to physician well-being. So, what did he say?

In the clinical area, Dr. Kirch believes that the ACA is likely to be modified but is here to stay long term. Although the ACA is good because it brings a lot of previously uninsured patients under the umbrella of health care, it is in itself also a stressor because of the administrative and clinical changes that are required within health systems as more ethnically diverse and low-income patients are able to receive care. He noted that the response to the complicated and changing federal and state requirements and general uncertainty has been increased consolidation within the marketplace. This consolidation is a major disruption, with more health systems, hospitals, and clinics involved in mergers. Dr. Kirch noted that these mergers are still primarily at the stage of anatomical but not physiological consolidation and will only be effective when they develop more values-based care and interprofessional teamwork. Simply getting larger does not mean greater efficiency. This rapid process of consolidation is leading to the disappearance of private practice, with surveys of current medical students showing that many expect to be career employees rather than running their own practices. Commenting on the way we now have to work, tied to our computers by so much required documentation, Dr. Kirch suggested that if aliens visited our hospitals today, they would think the main role of the physicians in white coats was to look after computers!

The second major disruption of the clinical environment is the aging of the Baby Boomers, sometimes thought of as a "silver tsunami," with 10,000 Boomers turning 65 years of age every day. Over the next few decades this will lead to a massive increase in older patients with chronic illnesses that will be a major workforce challenge, at the same time that physicians themselves are aging. It is estimated that by 2030 we will be short between 40,000 and 120,000 physicians nationally. The response to this shortage from Congress, as Dr. Kirch described, is to continue a "temporary" cap on residency places, which is now in its twenty-first consecutive year! Congress needs to wake up and stop limiting the number of residency places at a time of physician shortages and increasing population base and need.

Dr. Kirch described three other significant issues that will markedly disrupt the clinical environment, are very relevant to physician well-being and are discussed throughout this book, and must be resolved: the need for 1) more diversity within the health care professions, 2) organizational change to reduce burnout, and 3) improved medically driven leadership. His comments on the leadership issue are especially important; he sees a need for more assertive and better leadership to improve the health care system, with less focus on economic bottom lines and more on clinical and well-being outcomes for both patients and providers. As such, he believes that future leaders will be increasingly defined by their ability to actively listen and to be authentic, as is described several times through this book. A thick research resume will be less important to becoming a CEO or a dean than empathy, understanding, and communication skills.

The other two missions of most academic medical systems, and many physicians, are research and education. Both areas are open for disruption. Congress started this process in research with flat appropriations for the National Institutes of Health for a decade starting in 2006 until the past 4 years, which have been superinflationary. This now means that our national federal research funding has finally returned to the same inflation-adjusted level as 2006. Other countries, however, are putting a much larger share of their national product into scientific research and development, so the United States is drifting behind on this front. A more significant concern that Dr. Kirch noted is the increasingly antiscience mentality of the U.S. public and some politicians, reflected in the debates around climate change and vaccine safety. In this "post-truth" environment, feelings seem to count more than facts; such beliefs and attitudes may lead to reduced public emphasis on research in the future.

Regarding education, it is changing considerably, and both students and teachers have new preferences and perspectives. The major disruptive change here is technology, which also clearly disrupts both the clinical and research areas of health care. In medicine, knowledge doubles every few months, and these terabytes of information have overwhelmed the personal capacity of all physicians to keep up. This overload is causing a real paradigm shift at the educational level; it is no longer possible to fill doctors with enough facts to get the job done, as used to be the approach to medical education. An international move is being made for curricula to move away from the accumulation of facts toward the development of core competencies and skills that allow individual lifelong learners to teach themselves, using the "just in time" resources available when and where needed. In medical schools, the knowledge taught in the future will be considered foundational knowledge that will change over time, and more emphasis will be placed on non-knowledge-based competencies and skills, such as interprofessional practice, personal and professional development, critical thinking and reasoning, and interpersonal communication. Students are continuing to change their learning styles, and some schools may attempt to eliminate all formal lectures, moving to curricula that are more interactive and aided by technologies such as virtual reality.

Physicians—whatever their primary interests, be they clinical, research, educational, or administrative—are going to have to get used to a lot of changes in the future. These changes, or responses to the disruptive forces described here, need to be made with an eye on the health and well-being of physicians and other providers so as to not exacerbate their current stress-related problems.

I turn now to the current book, *Physician Well-Being: Cases and Solutions*, and how it can best be used. Although each chapter stands alone and the book can be read in any order, the text does follow several themes. The first chapter sets the scene and examines the current culture of medicine and the unintended consequences of professionalism. The "compulsive triad" of the doctor's personality—doubt, guilt, and an exaggerated sense of responsibility—works synergistically with the outdated ethical obligations of the Hippocratic Oath, which contains nothing about caring for oneself or other physicians. The chapter also examines the impact of the cultural implicit beliefs that result from this concept of professionalism, encouraging long hours of work that interfere with family relationships, and the effect of lawsuits on physicians' wellness and practices, leading to the conclusion that physicians need to treat themselves very differently in the future.

Chapters 2, 3, and 4 comprise scenarios in a large health system and a multidisciplinary clinic and focus strongly on solutions that work in typical current-day health environments. These range from the introduction of systemic changes that make clinician well-being a core outcome of future health systems, including the implementation and function of chief wellness officer positions, to organizational ways of reducing the stigma of psychiatric disorders and modifications to medical licensing systems. I describe change management processes at a patient-care level, including team care, mentorship, and improved efficiencies that reduce time-wasting administrative work and make effective use of technologies such as the EMR, telemedicine, and mobile devices. Finally, I discuss several approaches to support the individual resilience of clinicians.

Chapters 5, 6, and 7 focus on solutions needed to improve the onboarding of physicians in the early years of their career, starting first in pre-med before focusing on medical school and residency. Much of the problem we face is cultural, so change has to start early, before physicians are fully minted. Here I describe the impact of adverse childhood experiences, the medical school selection process, the style of board examinations, and the crushing debt levels, as well as the need and approach to combat implicit biases, especially in teaching faculty. Increasing the diversity of the medical workforce is essential so that we more closely mirror the patient populations we treat. Thus, I discuss gender and racial discrimination issues and solutions, as well as the need for formal well-being curricula in medical schools and residency programs. For those students and physicians who need treatment, whether it is by therapists, coaches, or psychiatrists, outcomes are known to be good once they are engaged in care, so the concept I propose of psychiatrists taking up the role of the "doctor's doctor" is a logical one.

In the final chapters, Chapters 8, 9, and 10, I focus on a broad variety of solutions, ranging from alternative medical careers, as well as nonclinical careers for some, to the use of technologies that allow us to work from anywhere, to how physicians can help combat climate change and improve the health not only of the planet and of their patients but also of themselves. I place a strong focus on medical marriages and how to make them work, especially when raising children in a shift-work environment, as well as on the eventual transition to retirement that many physicians dread but that is inevitable. In the final chapter, I describe how medical societies can support and enhance the well-being of physicians using a community-focused model that deserves to be implemented widely across the United States.

My intention is for this book to be read by, and useful to, any physicians and medical or pre-medical students as well as members of the general public. My hope is that it will highlight the professional mindset of most physicians and how this may interact with some of the stressors and illnesses that affect physicians and therefore potentially their patients. This book is about solutions for and changes to the culture and practice of medicine that need to be made so today's medical students and residents—impressive, intelligent, and committed people—can practice in a more forgiving environment than my generation has experienced. Countless other changes can be made that will improve the lives of future physicians, and I covered many of these, especially those relating to the treatment of physicians with psychiatric or substance-related disorders, in my first book, *Physician Suicide: Cases and Commentaries* (Yellowlees 2018), which can be read in tandem with this book with relatively little overlap.

Professionals from any discipline are driven by a combination of four sets of rewards for their work and careers, namely, the meaning and impact of their work, the opportunity for collegiality and friendships, and, of course, money and time. Physicians as a group do well with the first three drivers but poorly on the last; we do not have enough time to practice medicine properly or to spend on outside interests and with our families and loved ones. This must change so that physicians in future generations may have an overall improved sense of their own well-being.

Peter Yellowlees, MBBS, M.D.
Sacramento, California, June 2019

References

Yellowlees P: Physician Suicide: Cases and Commentaries. Washington, DC, American Psychiatric Association Publishing, 2018
Yellowlees P: Why is Physician Well-Being Declining? It's the System, Stupid. Medscape, September 6, 2019. Available at: https://www.medscape.com/viewarticle/917693. Accessed September 7, 2019.

ACKNOWLEDGMENTS

I WISH PRIMARILY TO acknowledge the interest and support throughout the writing of this book from my wife, Barb. She has made a major contribution to the writing of the book as my primary editor and literary critic. She has also listened to me and critiqued my ideas as I struggled to constantly improve the fictional cases I have included, ensuring that they remained both realistic and relevant and were focused on solutions that work in the real world. Little mention is made in the literature on physician health about the details of the daily events and pressures that contribute to the lifestyle of many physicians and that inadvertently lead to many unintended consequences of our professionalism. This book is an attempt to offer suggestions for change to the culture of medicine and the way that physicians practice their art, with the hope that it may improve the understanding of the lives of current generations of physicians and prevent further suffering in future generations and their loved ones.

I have worked with numerous dedicated people in the area of physician health during the past decade at the University of California (UC) Davis and wish to acknowledge all of them, whether they are mentioned by name here or not, as well as all my many physician patients. My recently retired departmental chair, Robert Hales, M.D., has always been very supportive of this interest, as has the team from the UC Davis Office of Medical Administration, including J. Douglas Kirk, M.D., and Leslie Navarra, in association with their other support staff. Jennifer Bannister, M.A., Michelle Burke-Parish, Ph.D., and Jerry Elder have been unfailingly helpful while I have worked with numerous faculty in my role as chief wellness officer and on the Medical Staff Well-Being Committee at UC Davis over the past 8 years. I wish to especially acknowledge Margaret Rea, Ph.D.; Katren Tyler, M.D.; Andres Sciolla, M.D.; Jessica Haskins, Ph.D.; Celia Chang, M.D.; Carol Kirshnit, Ph.D.; Debra Kahn, M.D.; Nasim Hedayati, M.D.; and Jeffrey Uppington, M.D.

Individuals who have helped me with collegiality, advice, and assistance as I have continuously learned about the many aspects of physician health include Jay Shore, M.D., and my colleagues at the other UC campuses: Karen Miotto, M.D.; Anju Hurria, M.D.; Thomas Savides, M.D.; and Diane Sliwka, M.D. Within California, I wish to acknowledge the leadership shown by the Sacramento Sierra Valley Medical Society, particularly Aileen Wetzel, Lindsay Coates, and Rajiv Misquitta, M.D. Finally, many expert papers and books are quoted and referenced throughout this book, and I thank all of these contributors who are so referenced.

I would also like to acknowledge the expertise and support of the team at American Psychiatric Association Publishing, who have been unfailingly helpful to me throughout the whole writing and publishing process. I would like to specifically mention Laura Roberts, M.D., John McDuffie, Jennifer Gilbreath, Greg Kuny, and Tammy Cordova.

Chapter 1

"OUR DEDICATED DAD"

Scenario

Robert and Belinda were shown into the unfamiliar corner office on the top floor of the hospital's old wing by a man in scrubs who introduced himself simply as Barry. They had never met Barry.

"You will need to clear out Dr. Richmond's closet by tomorrow at the latest, because the new surgeon starts this week, and we need to get her things moved in."

The three looked uncomfortably at each other for what felt like a long, awkward moment.

"What are we meant to go through?" asked Robert.

"Just the personal things your father kept locked in that large mahogany armoire. Here's the key, and feel free to use the boxes I left for you." Barry pointed to the stack of boxes as he moved toward the door. "I'm sorry about your dad, and I'm sorry that although I worked for him for so long, this is the first and probably the last time I will meet you. He was a great doctor. The patients really liked him. He sure put in long hours."

Robert and Belinda looked around the rather large and barren office, with its massive wooden desk. Nothing was on it, not a single pen or paper clip. Nothing. The two nonwindowed walls were covered with photos that their dad had apparently taken over decades but with no one they recognized. Catching their looks of confusion, Barry explained that the photos were probably a combination of staff and grateful former patients. Then he vanished down the hall, leaving Dr. Richmond's adult children somewhat chilled at the task before them. They could not help but notice the absence of family photos. Not a single photo of his son, his daughter, or his wife of more than 40 years. Their father, Dr. Paul Richmond, had died suddenly from a heart attack a few days before while he was preparing for a particularly challenging surgical case. His death had been a complete shock to everyone. No one had seen it coming, or so his family thought.

To let in more light, Belinda pulled the cord on the blinds, which brought down layers of dust. Evidently, they had not been opened in years, which seemed sad because once the blinds were opened, they could see a large park full of trees and walking paths across the parking lot.

"Let's pack up whatever we find and get out of here. We can let Mom decide what she wants to do with his stuff when we drop it off at her house. There can't really be much left here to go through." Robert turned to the armoire and used the key to open the door. A few papers slipped out, landing at his feet. The chest was packed full of papers and cards in every drawer and shelf, literally hundreds of old letters and cards dating back over many years. Robert tossed a stack to Belinda as he opened a card. It had been written 20 years earlier and was from the wife of a patient for whom his father had cared. The wife was full of grief at the loss of her husband but thanked their dad for giving her husband the extra 5 years no one else thought he would have. She also thanked him for being available 7 days a week and for all his outstanding care. Robert leafed through some more of the letters at random.

"Looks like his patients really did like him. There are so many cards and letters describing Dad's dedication, what a great doctor he was, and lots of comments about how much time he spent with them. So many write that Dad was always there for these people. That phrase keeps coming up. I should feel pride, but part of me is a little angry and sort of jealous." The brother and sister looked sadly at each other before agreeing to go through a few letters but then just pack it all up and get out.

After an hour, Belinda sighed. "I don't know the man whom all these people have written to. The way they describe him as so available, so warm, so caring—I guess it's nice that they seem to have gotten so much from our dad, but I'm kind of sad that we didn't have him around very much at home. He was home most nights, but usually too late to eat dinner with us, and he usually made morning rounds 7 days a week. With his job this may have been necessary, I guess, but most of his colleagues took turns making weekend rounds for each other so they had time off. I wonder why he didn't do that?"

Instead of leaving rapidly as they had planned, both just sat and continued reading the many documents, fascinated and curious.

"It's obvious he did a lot more than just treat patients," said Robert another hour later, looking up from the photo album he was perusing and glancing thoughtfully toward Belinda. "I've been surprised at all the extra work he did that we didn't know about. All the pressures on him over the course of his long career. It's interesting going through his papers, even though it's a rather strange experience being here without him. Dad's office always seemed off limits to us. I wonder if that was just what we thought. I don't recall him ever telling us we weren't welcome to visit him here. It's odd but sort of comforting to sit here, in his worn-out leather chair, peeking into chapters of his life we didn't know about. Somehow, I don't think he would mind, but I wish we had asked him about all of this when we had a chance. Reading these papers is giving me a completely different impression of Dad."

Belinda took a deep breath and put down the letter she was reading. "I know what you mean. Take this letter, for example. It's from a patient whom he seems to have operated on about 20 years ago. Dad was just so devoted to his patients, and it looks like they reciprocated. Let me read it to you."

Dear Dr. Richmond,

I am writing to thank you for all the care you gave me and for saving my life not once, but three times. You were constantly available for me and must have almost lived in the hospital when I was your patient, especially when I had complication after complication. You were so concerned for me through my three emergency surgeries. I am sure that many of your patients must thank you for the extraordinary work that you do, and I am proud to be one of them. I know I wasn't always easy to deal with.

Your nurses are wonderful and caring too. I bet you don't know that they talk about you as though you walk on water. They talk about working on "RW," by which they mean "Richmond Ward," although I know the signs say Ward 3A. They always talk about you very respectfully, always calling you Dr. Richmond, although they have nicknames for some of the other doctors. I understand why they respect you so much. You are more than a great surgeon; you are simply kind and always there for your patients. Thank you for answering my long list of questions and letting me feel safe to ask you anything. Thank you for never making me feel rushed.

Thank you for all your expert care and attention. I don't know how you manage to do it, but you do, and I appreciate it.

Sincerely,

Thelma Close

Belinda brushed a tear from her eye as she laid down the letter. She caught a glimpse of herself in the wall mirror; the university logo embroidered on her gray sweatshirt caught her eye, and she remembered her first day on campus when her parents dropped her off for her freshman year. The last item her dad had picked up for her at the bookstore checkout was that sweatshirt. She knew she hadn't even thanked him. This was still her go-to sweatshirt after all these years. How she wished she had thanked him! Belinda's thick blonde hair complemented her blue eyes. She had the same color hair and eyes as her dad. She looked at her reflection and was grateful that she still took her daily run, which kept her fit and healthy. She choked up a little, remembering a few times she had complained to her dad that he didn't come run with her. She knew she had resented his not taking time to enjoy the fresh air and get in an early morning run, but she was beginning to understand why he hadn't taken time for himself. He put his patients first.

"You know, it's so hard reading all these letters. There are literally hundreds of them from patients and colleagues over the years. I think he must have kept almost everything that was ever written to or about him throughout his whole career. The dreadful irony is that he was the only one who knew about all of these wonderful letters and citations." She paused. "And we are only seeing them because of his sudden death last week. Just 58 years of age. He kept all this stuff in this office, filed neatly away. I don't think Mom knows anything about these letters and how his patients felt about him. It almost feels like we are breaking into a separate part of his life—the world where he worked. I feel like we're intruders into a huge part of his life that he kept private from us. He must have known we would see this someday."

Robert listened to all Belinda said. He was feeling distressed by the experience of going through their father's office. Robert Richmond looked very much like his father had when he was 30—the same swept-back blonde hair, already beginning to show silver strands. His face was less worn and beaten than his father's had been at this age, a result of being less sleep deprived than his dad had been. Robert's chosen profession was economics; he was fast becoming well known for creating algorithms to explain the economic relationship between poverty and climate change. He had never regretted his career choice, although he knew his dad had been disappointed that he hadn't gone to medical school.

He responded to Belinda. "Frankly, it's weird—us finding out so much about him at this time. I must have read 20 other letters like that one. Part of me is proud that his patients adored him so, but part of me is just mad at him for what we went through. While he gave so much of himself to his patients, we had an absent father whom we are only really getting to know now that it's too late. He's gone. And to make the irony even worse, to die in his operating room just a few weeks before he was finally meant to slow down! He had been planning the perfect retirement, would finally spend more time with Mom doing all the things they have put off over the years because of his devotion to work. He'd worked hard to save enough to allow an early retirement. It's all so confusing. I have had such mixed feelings about him for many years, and now my uncertainty is made worse by finding all this stuff, having to sort through all of his professional belongings. I have to say, Belinda, that I think we drew the short straw, having to do this job. I would rather be going over the finances or sorting out his clothes and other belongings at home with Mom. But someone has to do this, and I think it would be really hard on Mom right now."

He sat back and looked out of the office window, then glanced at his father's beautiful oak desk with the surgical society's painted coat of arms carved into its base. Stylish glass mementos of conferences attended in India and Chile, embossed with his father's name and the year they had been given, sat proudly on a shelf by the door. Robert looked around the room that had been so central to his father's existence, where he had spent so much time and seen many of his patients. His father had not done much to decorate the office beyond the walls of photographs. Only a bare minimum of furniture occupied the space—the desk and his chair, plus three chairs for visitors. The armoire they were slowly emptying also contained numerous awards, transcripts, and membership certificates of his father's many degrees and academic qualifications, along with some favorite historical surgical prints and photographs of various major professional events. It seemed sad and disappointing that he had hidden the evidence of his successful career. Their father had always been modest, but it was odd that these were not on display. Perhaps he had just never gotten around to having them framed and hung.

Robert realized that in a matter of days the documentation of his dad's career would be gone, and a new surgeon would move into this office. He wondered what the point had been of his dad keeping all these mementos, letters, inscribed books, and photos. He was pretty sure that his father had not gone through them himself and that most were just filed away. So, what did they show, and what could they learn about their father's life from them?

As Robert contemplated their father's private study, Belinda continued to read through the files. Like her brother, she also had avoided going into a health profession, despite her parents' quiet pressure to do so. She had gotten a master's degree in business administration (MBA) and was now working for a startup business that created and sold a new line of easy-to-use garden hoses, and it was expanding rapidly. She turned to her brother and realized that, as usual, he was thinking deeply about their task and would tend to see most of the negatives involved in it. She knew her role, as the more outgoing of the Richmond siblings, was to keep him positive and not allow him to be too inwardly focused, an attribute she had also seen in their father. She looked across at Robert and tried to bring him out of his reverie.

"Don't look so upset, Robert. We will get through all of this today, and whatever papers we can't sort out here, we'll just take to Mom's house. Let's make sure we learn as much about Dad as we can and take advantage of this opportunity. I'm glad we have this chance to find out so much about him. He never talked about work very much. In fact, he didn't seem to talk about himself much at all. He was more interested in finding out how we were doing at school or whatever we were up to. You must admit, we were always loved and supported by him. We just didn't seem to have much time to have fun with him. He made sure we could try any sport we wanted, even though he didn't come see us compete. It's too bad he didn't take time for golf or tennis. He didn't seem to take time for himself much."

Robert nodded. "I was just thinking, what was the point of Dad keeping all this paraphernalia? It was only meaningful to him, and is much less important to us, and at the end of the day we'll throw a lot of it away, unless Mom wants any of it. I don't know what I expected to find here. Interestingly, most of the cards and letters are from many years ago. Maybe patients send thankful e-mails nowadays. But something did surprise me: that whole drawer of letters and correspondence he kept that concerned his contacts with the various hospitals, insurance companies, malpractice companies, and medical boards he was involved with over the years. Some of those letters are quite remarkable and show how much pressure he was under during his professional life. That was a real eye-opener to me."

Belinda nodded. "He was under so much pressure during his career, and yet he was resilient and was able to push back. Some of the nonsense he had to put up with from these other groups amazes me. His ability to fight back on behalf of what he thought was right, and what seems to have usually been in the best interest of his patients, is a whole new part of Dad that I just didn't know about. No wonder he used to sometimes complain about administrators not understanding the stress he was under. I can't seem to find support from the people he worked with. He really had some huge pressures, and I feel guilty for not understanding that before."

"Did you look at all the letters from his malpractice company about that lawsuit he mentioned to us at home a few times over the years?" Robert asked.

"Yes. Incredible, aren't they? I haven't read them in detail yet, but the simple volume of communications with all the lawyers is shocking." Belinda paused. "There's such a contrast between what he told us and what was actually happening. He minimized it totally at home and even made a joke of it at times. Do you remember how he used to say how he wished he had implanted the fishing nets we saw on vacations into his hernia patients rather than the artificial mesh implants he used that led to the lawsuit against him? I wonder if Mom knows what was really happening and how much time and effort it must have taken him to defend himself. Looking at the paperwork, it must have taken Dad hours and hours of time to respond over a decade of legal arguments and fights. It looks like you've read more of the details than I did; did you really work out why he was sued and what happened at the end in court, when he won the case? He may have won the lawsuit, but it seems like he paid a huge price for it with all the years of his time and money it took to finally win."

"Yes, I have," Robert answered. "But it's hard to work out the details just from the paperwork. I wish Dad was still here so we could understand all this better, and how it affected him. As far as I can see, multiple lawsuits were filed against the artificial mesh manufacturers and against the doctors like Dad who had implanted them. And then there were some other suits against Dad from individual patients, separate from the class-action suits, for specific damages they believed they had personally suffered from the surgeries, especially for what seems to be called 'pain and suffering.' We'll never understand what happened. We're only seeing pieces.

"It's actually the letters about some of those individual lawsuits that are the most interesting. Some of the patients seem to have been claiming really substantial disabilities, such as permanent severe abdominal pain that stopped them being able to sit comfortably, or chronic migraines and loss of employment. And they all claimed that he was negligent for using the hernia mesh in his clinical trials, even though it had been fully tested and approved by the federal authorities, and they had signed consents for him to use the implants. The letters I found most painful to read were the ones he wrote to his insurance company defending what he had done and responding to the individual patient claims, some of which just seemed so unlikely. He seemed to have been trying to walk a tightrope—defending himself and his clinical practice while at the same time not wanting to disrespect the claims of the patients. Did you see the claim from that patient who said that one of the nurses had given him an injection in the wrong place, which had led to chronic nerve pain in his leg? She was suing Dad for overseeing poor care after her operation, even though in that case the mesh implant seemed to have worked perfectly. I could sense Dad's frustration at being sued for something he had no control over."

Belinda began to realize the enormous burden her dad had carried for more than a decade. He had gone through it pretty much alone. No one in the family had known what he was dealing with. No one could help support him.

"He wrote letters about this for more than a decade," she said. "And he finally had to go to court about 5 years ago. I think I finally understand why he became so cynical about research and why he stopped doing clinical trials in the last 10 years or so. Did you see that letter he wrote to the other implant manufacturer he worked with, withdrawing from doing any more clinical trials, despite having worked closely with them for many years? That really changed his life in the second part of his career, because it meant that he didn't go to so many conferences to present his findings, and it took a great interest out of his professional life. I had never realized until now that these lawsuits most likely led him to withdraw from his research career. That must have been a great loss for him. I guess he decided that it was just not worth it. I'm going to sit Mom down when we get home tonight and try to find out how much she knew about all this. I wonder if he kept her in the dark most of the time, and if she didn't know much more about it than we did. What was it that led him to keep so much to himself? I wish he could have shared some of this with us, if only to get it off his chest."

"I agree," said Robert. "At one level, talking to him was always frustrating because he would just minimize any problems and say everything was fine. If he didn't want to talk about something, he simply was not going to. And the lawyers telling him not to talk to anyone about the cases would have made it worse. It was as though he had a coat of armor on the whole time that stopped anyone from trying to find out what was happening inside of him in his work and professional life. I wonder if he was a typical doctor in that respect. Are they all trained to keep their stresses inside? Maybe they think they can't acknowledge any weaknesses because if they did, the metaphorical walls would fall down, and the whole castle of the medical culture would collapse?"

"I don't know," said Belinda. "Maybe that whole approach helped him survive the pressures of his profession. Whatever else, it is really remarkable how strong he seemed to be and how he coped with this sort of stress on top of all the pressures of his usual clinical practice, while at the same time not sharing his concerns with us, or likely with anyone except maybe his lawyer, from the look of some of his letters. Now it's too late to help him. I feel torn, because we could have been there for him, but he shut us out. He probably thought he could manage and not lean on us, but his good intentions led to his becoming more isolated over the years. I saw a book on mindfulness in the armoire, but it doesn't look as though he read it. It seems his whole life was dedicated to helping everyone except himself."

She shook her head. "You know, this is getting a bit morbid. I miss Dad so much. I just wish I had spent more time with him and that he had carved out more time for us. All those weekends we could have done things. All the family holidays interrupted. His insistence that he had to go to the hospital and round on his patients at Christmas and Thanksgiving—taking so much longer than he would say. It always felt to me that our family celebrations inevitably took second place. I don't remember anyone complaining to him about late dinners. Maybe he didn't realize the toll it took on us."

Robert looked over at his sister, lifting his head out of a file marked *Resident Teaching*. "You know, Belinda, I will always miss Dad and wish we had spent more time with him. I've been going through paper copies of his surgery lectures to his residents in this file. It was just so typical of him to always keep a hard copy of everything he did—he never really did trust computers. We both know that he had a really dry sense of humor, but we saw it so rarely. Looking at some of his lectures, I'm surprised to see how much humor he threaded quite well throughout them. He was really funny. He used lots of hilarious cartoons, especially those of *The New Yorker* style. I remember him telling me how proud he was that he had been given the residents award as 'teacher of the year' on three occasions in recent years, and I can see now how he did it. His lectures look like stories, only they are stories of patients and clinical settings, beautifully illustrated and both funny and thoughtful. It must have taken him ages to make up these PowerPoint presentations. Somehow, they remind me of the sort of surgeon he apparently was—careful, thoughtful, and sensitive to the needs of his patients and all who worked with him. You should definitely go through some of these lectures to look at how his personality shone through, even when discussing how to take out a gallbladder or repair a bowel."

"Maybe, but I'm not sure I really want to see the detailed photos!" Belinda laughed. "Not my scene, and never will be. But that's interesting to hear, because I really hadn't realized how much teaching he was doing, especially recently. I know he used to have those Christmas parties each year at home for all the residents when we were kids, but I've always thought that was because we had a large house that was close to the hospital. Now that I have my own family, I realize what a commitment that was for both Dad and Mom, because a lot of work was involved in getting everything just right for the party, and I remember how proud Dad was of his barbecue skills. I haven't ever really thought of Dad as a teacher. He really enjoyed having the residents over for the annual parties; I wonder why they stopped having them."

Robert interjected. "One thing this reminds me of, and that I will never forget, is that amazing conference he took all of us to, the whole family, when he was president of the state surgical society, and he had to give the main conference keynote speech. He had us sit up in front with Mom in the reserved seats, and I was so proud when he came onto the stage. All the house lights were dimmed, and just a single flood light followed him on the stage. He looked wonderful in his pinstripe suit and that blue tie mom gave him. I remember being surprised by how great he looked, and how the entire audience clapped for him for so long. He just stood there before us giving his speech, taking his time, and smiling at us in the front row. I remember thinking 'that's my dad'—I almost couldn't believe he was on that stage, with everyone anxious to hear him speak. In retrospect, that must have been one of the highlight events of his professional life. I'm sorry we didn't think to celebrate with him that night. As I remember, you and I went out for pizza by ourselves. We didn't think to invite Dad or Mom." He paused. "Not many children get to see their fathers like that. We were so lucky having him as a dad in many ways. I wonder if he has any photos around here from that night? It seems odd there are no family photos here in his office."

Belinda went back to the armoire, where she took out several thick files marked *Hospital Administration*. "I saw these files earlier and didn't think they would be too exciting. How about I go through them quickly? We'll probably be throwing most of them out." She carried the files over to her father's desk and spread them out so that she could review each of them separately. She moved the large metal wastebasket close to the edge of the desk so she could rapidly read, sort, and discard the voluminous papers. Robert remained sitting in one of the comfortable patient chairs, reading files of academic papers and correspondence to his father, discarding most of them. After a few minutes he looked up, because he noticed Belinda had stopped filling her wastebasket. To his surprise, she was reading papers from the first file in detail. She was frowning and staring intently at what she was reviewing. Her right hand was on her forehead, and she was concentrating deeply.

"What's going on?" Robert said. "I thought these files would be quick and easy."

"So did I," said Belinda. "But they're fascinating, and I'm learning so much more about the pressures on Dad, things he never told us about. It's remarkable what he went through. Do you remember a few years ago, when he was chief of staff? I certainly didn't appreciate how much he was responsible for managing. It seems he was in that position for 2 years, as well as being deputy chief for 2 years beforehand. Remember, he told us that it was just a part-time role that he did on a voluntary basis? It was so much more. That job ended up being something that almost took over his whole professional life for several years. You and I were both away at college, and we used to worry about how Mom was always home alone. Dad was at work so much. He would come home after 8 P.M. most nights and seemed to work most weekends. We were really worried about both of them. Dad was working crazy hours and telling us he was doing lots of extra surgeries because they were short of doctors, while Mom was just sad and lonely all the time. You have to read these files after me, because they explain exactly what was going on. I can't believe he never even mentioned all of these issues, when it looks like they took over his life for a long time. How on Earth did he manage to cope with all the pressures?"

Robert looked puzzled. "What pressures? What was happening?"

"Well, I haven't read everything yet, of course, but it looks like the hospital's CEO[1] and his financial officer were fired on the same day, with no notice. It seems that when Dad was chief of staff, he wanted to employ much-needed additional physicians and nurses because the

---

[1]CEO = chief executive officer.

hospital was constantly full to overflowing, but the CEO kept refusing, saying they couldn't afford it. Dad didn't believe the hospital was unable financially to manage hiring the staff he was requesting. The hospital was always so full. So Dad went through the accounts and discovered that hundreds of thousands of dollars seemed to be missing, and then he confronted the CEO.

"From the look of these letters, the CEO actually tried to fire Dad, calling him a 'troublemaker' in the letter I just read. Here's Dad's response." She paused as she continued reading. "He refused to get upset about the name calling and also refused to resign, saying it was his role as chief of staff to help all the clinical staff, and if that meant fighting to increase their numbers as needed clinically, then he would continue to do that. At the end of the letter, he formally requested an independent external audit of the hospital finances over the previous decade. Dad sent copies to all members of the hospital board and the executive committee. That was gutsy of him. It must have been all-out war. I can't believe we didn't know anything about all of this, although I do now recall a couple of articles being written in the local newspaper about the eventual sudden resignation of the hospital CEO and CFO.[2]"

"Would you pass me the letters you've already read?" asked Robert. "It sounds like Dad must have eventually won this battle, but what a nightmare! I can't believe he was threatened with being fired. Dad was the most ethical and honest man I've ever known. That is one area I have always tried to copy. He would never do anything that he thought was wrong, so it must have been unbelievably painful for him to be in that position, essentially an internal whistleblower against someone in a more senior administrative position. And it doesn't sound like he had a lot of support, at least initially. I suddenly understand why he was never at home and why he and mom were constantly worried that his job was at risk. If Dad had ever been fired, it would have been total humiliation for him, whatever the reasons and the situation. He lived his life to be a highly respected doctor. Thank goodness he managed to survive such an awful situation. I guess we'll never really know what sort of long-term toll these events took on him."

"You're right," said Belinda, "although it does explain one of the attitudes he had in the later years of his career. I had a long talk with him a few years ago about leadership when I was applying for a new job. He was very interesting on the topic. I argued that I could easily move from

---

[2]CFO = chief financial officer.

one industry to another if I had good generic leadership skills, and at that stage I was thinking of doing just that. A great job had opened up at a major software company, and as you know, I am not great with computers. He had a very different view. He told me he believed that if a high level of technical knowledge was required in the industry I was moving into, then I should get that knowledge first. Interestingly, he used health care as an example. He said there had been a move in the past 20 or 30 years for nonphysicians with MBAs to increasingly take up CEO and other health care leadership positions, and he felt that his generation of doctors had let control of the health system slip away from them. He made it clear to me that he felt strongly that leaders in an industry as complicated as health care should have been clinicians of some sort at one time, so that they truly understood the pressures of clinical practice. I guess that explains why the new CEO of the medical center, whom Dad was involved in appointing, was a physician administrator. And it probably at least partly explained why Dad was prepared to take on the role of chief of staff. He would have seen it as being his duty and the right thing to do."

Robert agreed. "Yes, Dad was always ruled by his sense of duty. If he had a problem, his answer was just to work harder until he succeeded. It's fascinating finding out all these extra things about his work life, and it's amazing how he coped with the pressures on top of his patient load. But there was a cost for dad, as we both know. While you were reading all the legal papers about the fraud case, I found a plain file in the bottom drawer of his desk. It's not marked on the outside in any way, and knowing Dad, it's really rather sad. It's full of old holiday brochures that he had read and notated. They go back about 20 years, brochures from countries all over the world, and quite a few are about adventure tours for couples, like safaris, hiking, boating, and cycling. You know how he was going to retire in a few months, and he and mom have been planning a number of trips that they would take once he had stopped work. Well, it looks to me like he'd been thinking of these trips for many years. It's such a shame that he worked so hard and so selflessly all his life and didn't get to take those trips. He and Mom have always taken annual holidays, but usually around the family. It looks like he had a whole lot of other plans or ideas that never happened."

"I wonder if he ever even discussed these vacation plans with Mom," Belinda responded. "I still can't believe he died just before he retired. He spent his entire life taking care of others, but he didn't take time for himself, let alone Mom. And now he's gone, so suddenly, and with no warning."

Over the next hour, Robert and Belinda continued looking through their father's files, throwing out most items. They were exhausted and had become subdued, talking less and less as the day dragged on. They seemed to be getting near to the end, with only a few files left to review, when Belinda suddenly sat up, holding a letter in her hand and staring at it with her eyes wide open. She clenched the paper tightly, as though she could not believe what she was reading, and looked at Robert, who was regarding her in surprise. She burst into tears.

"Oh, Robert, I don't believe this." She forced the words out in a faltering voice. "It looks like Dad had heart problems for years and did nothing about them. Look at this letter! It's dated a month before his death. Come here and take a look; tell me I'm wrong. I think his death could have been prevented!" She sank down into the desk chair again as the impact of the letter hit home. "This letter makes it pretty clear that Dad was not taking any heed of longstanding cardiac symptoms. He seems to have known he was at risk, but he just put off seeking the care he needed. Why didn't he seek help himself?"

Robert slowly got up from his chair, looking suddenly pale and troubled. He moved to the desk to read the letter Belinda was holding and had to pry it from her hands. The letterhead was that of a long-term friend and colleague of his father's.

Dear Paul,

I decided to write to you personally after our discussions over the past several months and years, because I am most concerned about your health. I feel it necessary to document my concerns in the hope that you will follow up with my recommendations, which you have to this point refused to do. You are not physically invulnerable, and I believe you are in danger of having a heart attack or a stroke. I am aware that you do not have a primary care provider and have ordered all your own tests yourself, coming to see me only for a second opinion on your self-diagnosis. I would normally have written this letter to your primary care physician, copied to you, in the hope that they could persuade you to receive treatment.

I confirm that I have examined you on two occasions recently and that I agreed with your impression that the tight chest pain you have been getting for several years was most likely mild angina, getting worse over time. Your electrocardiograms have shown increasingly marked ischemic changes suggesting likely coronary artery obstruction by significant plaques in your left anterior descending artery, and possibly in other coronary arteries. Your lab work looks normal.

I informed you at our most recent consultation a month ago that you should be receiving medication treatment, including aspirin and beta-blockers, and that you should have an urgent angiogram, which could possibly lead to coronary stenting or coronary bypass surgery. You told me that you would think about this but made it clear that you also were busy, with lots of surgeries booked, and that you thought you would be fine until you retired next June as long as you took things slowly. You will recall that I asked if I could phone your wife about your condition, and you refused me permission.

Since that time, my nurses have tried numerous times to schedule your angiogram, and I have personally spoken to you twice on the phone to entreat you to seek urgent treatment to avoid a possible heart attack or stroke. This letter is the only approach beyond speaking to you that I can think of to try and get you to agree to what I believe is essential testing and treatment. Please do follow up with me urgently so that we can arrange these investigations and start you on appropriate treatment.

Yours truly,

Benjamin Scott, M.D.
Cardiologist

Commentary

The story of Paul Richmond, a widely respected and dedicated surgeon who gave his all, is not atypical of the stories of many highly successful and professional physicians over the past century. Dr. Richmond was, from the outside and from the perspective of his patients and colleagues, almost the stereotype of a wonderful, caring physician: always available, always caring, always professional—and seemingly invulnerable, able to cope with all sorts of stresses and pressures with apparently no substantial impact on himself. A picture of medical resiliency. This is just the type of picture that many physicians, not surprisingly, want to project to their patients, their families, and their communities, and most physicians can manage this act successfully, because to a great extent it is an act that has required a lot of training to develop and much concentration to maintain. So, let us now turn to the unintended consequences of professionalism in the context of the culture of medicine.

One of the interesting aspects of medicine is the implicit set of beliefs, ethics, values, and moral underpinnings associated with the culture of medicine. Dr. Joan Anzia, M.D., a psychiatrist from Northwestern University who has examined these in detail, presented her findings at the conference of the American College of Psychiatrists in February 2019. She described the following implicit beliefs as characterizing the culture of medicine (Anzia 2019):

- I can do without sleep.
- I don't have time to exercise.
- I eat and drink when I can.
- I can always do more. I can get it done.
- I have to do it perfectly or it's a personal failure.
- I can't tell anyone if and when I have doubts or vulnerabilities.
- If I ask for help, my colleagues won't trust or respect me.
- I'll just work even harder and keep everything under control. It'll be okay. I can't say no.

Dr. Anzia contrasted these beliefs with the needs of a culture of re-silience and wellness, which she noted includes

- Getting adequate sleep, exercise, nutrition, and hydration
- Accepting that doing everything is not possible but that the most im-portant and essential things should be done
- Understanding that, while doing your best, we are all humans, and perfection is impossible
- Isolating oneself from friends and colleagues is bad, and asking for help and advice is good
- Trying to have everything under rigid control is not good for anyone

Challenging these implicit beliefs is vitally important, and it needs to occur as early as possible, certainly through medical school. Unfortu-nately, many of these beliefs are hardwired into physicians trained over the past 30 years and are going to take a long time to change. They are driven by what Gabbard (1985) described as the "compulsive triad" of the doctor's personality—doubt, guilt, and an exaggerated sense of re-sponsibility, working synergistically with the ethical obligations of the Hippocratic Oath, which, while covering many positive aspects, con-tains nothing about self-care or the care of other physicians.

It is self-evident how this culture of medicine, driven by implicit be-liefs, promotes a sense of perfectionism such that any discovery of burn-out, or any deficit in professional behavior, is met with shame and denial by both the suffering physician and medical leaders. Dr. Anzia suggested that it may help to reconfigure the ethical principles on which all doctors depend. She recommended multiple changes to core ethical principles, many of which are included in the Hippocratic Oath doctors take at the end of medical school. A current-day version of the Hippo-cratic Oath as sworn by today's medical students at their commence-ment ceremony, taken from the University of California, Davis School of Medicine student handbook, is as follows (Health Professions Advising 2018):

> I swear to fulfill, to the best of my ability and judgment, this covenant:
>
> I will respect the hard-won scientific gains of those physicians in whose steps I walk, and gladly share such knowledge as is mine with those who are to follow.
>
> I will apply, for the benefit of the sick, all measures which are required, avoiding those twin traps of overtreatment and therapeutic nihilism.
>
> I will remember that there is art to medicine as well as science, and that warmth, sympathy, and understanding may outweigh the surgeon's knife or the chemist's drug.
>
> I will not be ashamed to say "I know not," nor will I fail to call in my colleagues when the skills of another are needed for a patient's recovery.
>
> I will respect the privacy of my patients, for their problems are not disclosed to me that the world may know. Most especially must I tread with care in matters of life and death. If it is given me to save a life, all thanks. But it may also be within my power to take a life; this awesome responsibility must be faced with great humbleness and awareness of my own frailty. Above all, I must not play at God.
>
> I will remember that I do not treat a fever chart, a cancerous growth, but a sick human being, whose illness may affect the person's family and economic stability. My responsibility includes these related problems, if I am to care adequately for the sick.
>
> I will prevent disease whenever I can, for prevention is preferable to cure.
>
> I will remember that I remain a member of society, with special obligations to all my fellow human beings, those sound of mind and body as well as the infirm.
>
> If I do not violate this oath, may I enjoy life and art, respected while I live and remembered with affection thereafter. May I always act so as to preserve the finest traditions of my calling and may I long experience the joy of healing those who seek my help.

What changes does Dr. Anzia suggest? She focuses on the ethical principles identified in the Oath and suggests changes as follows:

- *Beneficence* should include the principle that physicians must take care of their own bodies, minds, and spirits, and those of their colleagues and trainees, in order to do good for others.
- *Hope and optimism*: These principles have traditionally been interpreted as "for the patient" but could be fostered throughout medical training and practice as a value to help physicians.
- *Practice within the limits of competence* could be expanded to include the need for physicians to monitor themselves and their colleagues

in a team environment, looking for external or internal stressors that need changing.

- *Nonmaleficence* should be not only for patients but also for our colleagues and ourselves. Individual physicians and physician leadership should speak out when they see adverse impacts from, for example, the workplace environment.
- *Justice:* Physicians need adequate resources and time to look after themselves and their colleagues so that they can continue to perform at the top of their licenses.
- *Veracity* means speaking honestly about needed changes in our work.
- *Fidelity* means being faithful to oneself and one's own moral attitudes in order to practice effectively. Interestingly, some are trying to redefine burnout as a "moral injury" and have a good point about it at this deeply personal level.

The unintended consequences of the culture of medicine for Dr. Richmond were personal, in terms of his absence from home and distancing from his family and friends, his loss of time for lifestyle interests and passions outside of medicine, and his tragic, untimely, and potentially preventable death just before he was to retire and fulfill his long-held plans to travel with his wife. The long hours of work that physicians are trained to accept needs to be questioned, and this is a recurring theme throughout this book. What other profession in the twenty-first century could think that limiting resident work to a maximum of 80 hours per week could be seen as rational? The effects of overwork in junior doctors are brilliantly described in Kay's (2017) heartbreaking bestselling book detailing his work as a resident, which should be mandatory reading for all training directors and those involved in supporting inhumane hours of work for trainee physicians. In what other professions are incumbents proud of their often 7-day accessibility and of their capacity to perform physically arduous and demanding technical work such as surgery for shifts of more than 12 hours at a time? It is hardly surprising that physicians get used to working long hours, when so many go through an absurd baptism of fire otherwise called a residency program. The results of these unintended consequences for Dr. Richmond's wife and family were perhaps even greater than for him, as seen in Robert and Belinda's conversation: he was, to them and their mother, a lifelong physically—and often psychologically—absent father and husband. The only people not adversely affected by his professionalism and work practices were his patients, so it is not surprising they placed him on a psychological pedestal. This, of course, is part of the reward that many doctors seek, either consciously or unconsciously, and that keeps them working excessively throughout their careers.

The need to change the culture of medicine is also a major topic in my previous book, which focused on physician suicide. Several discussions focus on the ethical principles underpinning medicine and how these drive much of medical practice (Yellowlees 2018). Much of the current book is about how physicians, as inherently very resilient individuals, can overcome, avoid, or prevent these unintended consequences. My argument, however, is that although being resilient is very important for all physicians, and that resilience techniques can be successfully taught, it is not generally possible to "resilience yourself" out of highly stressful situations. Organizational, systemic, and culture change usually is required in many environments where physician stress or burnout is highly prevalent, as described in a comprehensive *NEJM Catalyst* (2018) collection of papers published in late 2018. Many approaches to reduce the impact of the more than 70 individual and external factors adversely affecting clinician well-being are also described by the impressive work of the National Academy of Medicine (2019), and the first change that has to happen is for physicians as a profession to learn that it is not necessary to sacrifice oneself on the altar of wildly excessive hours of work.

Another important theme in this scenario is the psychological defenses typically used by doctors—denial and intellectualization—as well as the issue of delayed gratification, putting off fun or joyful events, such as Dr. Richmond's travel, in deference to immediate work priorities, as described in Yellowlees (2018). These defenses are also sensitively discussed by Elton (2018), who has written a fascinating book focused on the inner lives of doctors that describes the psychological dynamics of many physicians whom she has treated in her psychological practice.

Dr. Richmond also experienced other major sources of stress common for many doctors, including being sued, which in some specialties such as obstetrics-gynecology is almost inevitable during the course of the average career, and interacting with nonclinical health care leaders who may have differing priorities or experiences and a much stronger focus on financial rather than clinical outcomes. The issue of health care leadership itself is very important for most doctors, but it also creates tremendous ambivalence in many potentially excellent medical leaders because it often requires gradual, almost complete cessation of clinical practice, something most doctors find very difficult to accept. This is discussed in more detail in Chapter 2. The final tragic topic in Dr. Richmond's scenario is how he treated himself, and did so inadequately, rather than putting himself in the role of patient and seeing a doctor for his own medical problems. About one-third of doctors are like Dr. Richmond and do not have a primary care physician, so they are unable to receive the regular medical care throughout their lives that all patients are advised to seek.

What, then, is the stereotype of the ideal doctor, and what do many pre-medical students fantasize that they will eventually become? The first point to make about this is that the topic is very popular and that perceptions of idealized physicians vary enormously. When I put "physician stereotypes" into Google, the search returned more than two million results, with the top pages primarily focused on humor or Hollywood's perceptions of doctors as seen through many popular television shows and movies that are now part of our culture. Although *Grey's Anatomy*, *Scrubs*, and *House*, all featuring doctors with various personal and interpersonal problems, have taken over from Marcus Welby, James Kildare, and Hawkeye Pierce, it is fair to say that most doctors, certainly those of Dr. Richmond's vintage, were more influenced by the physician representations of the twentieth century and see these as being their idealizations. These older, more professional versions of physicians are certainly what the bulk of today's medical profession would prefer as models for future physicians. It will be interesting to see if public perceptions of doctors change over time because of the influence of the current generation of TV doctors. Tanenbaum (2011) wrote an interesting article tracing the "25 Most Memorable TV Doctors," for those who wish to review the changing media perceptions of physicians.

What, then, are the professional attributes expected from physicians that Dr. Richmond demonstrated? And what is the nature of professionalism as it relates to the medical profession? These are core questions of interest to the Alpha Omega Alpha Honor Medical Society, which, with more than 40,000 active physician and medical student members, has recently published a comprehensive monograph on professionalism best practices in the modern era (Byyny et al. 2017). They noted that the practice of medicine is, at its core, dependent on a "covenant of trust," which is a contract that medical professionals have with patients and society that "determines medicine's values and responsibilities in the care of the patient and improving public health." They described the physician's side of the contract as follows:

> It starts with physicians understanding their obligations and commitments to serve and care for people, especially those who are suffering. Physicians must put patients first and subordinate their own interests to those of others. They should also adhere to high ethical and moral standards and a set of medical professional values. These values start with the precept of "do no harm." They include a simple code of conduct that explicitly states: no lying, no stealing, no cheating, and no tolerance for those who do. The Golden Rule, or ethic of reciprocity, common to many cultures throughout the world—"one should treat others as one would like others to treat oneself"—should be the ethical code or moral basis for how we treat each other. (Byyny et al. 2017, p. ix)

Dr. Richmond clearly upheld his side of this contract, even if he subordinated his own interests too much, something many physicians do. Changing this practice is something physicians need to consider in order to gain more balance in their lives in a way that does not disrupt patient care. Dr. Richmond certainly met the standard for professionalism described succinctly by the Royal College of Physicians and Surgeons of Canada in 2000, who defined the professional requirements of physicians as being the delivery of "the highest quality of care with integrity, honesty and compassion." They also noted that physicians "should be committed to the health and well-being of individuals and society through ethical practice, professionally led regulation, and high personal standards of behavior" (Royal College of Physicians and Surgeons of Canada 2016).

Along similar lines, the American College of Physicians in 2002 developed a physician charter that had three core principles (ABIM Foundation et al. 2002), namely

1. The primacy of patient welfare, or dedication to serving the interest of the patient, and the importance of altruism and trust
2. Patient autonomy, including honesty and respect for the patients' desire to make decisions about their care
3. Social justice, to eliminate discrimination in health care for any reason

In reviewing many of these issues, the Alpha Omega Alpha monograph described the professional core values that are typically included within the physician's oath all new doctors take and that underlie the professional behavior of most physicians throughout their professional lives, including the commitment to (Byyny et al. 2017, p. xi)

- Adhere to high ethical and moral standards—do right, avoid wrong, and do no harm.

- Subordinate personal interests to those of the patient.
- Avoid business, financial, and organizational conflicts of interest.
- Honor the social contract with patients and communities.
- Understand the nonbiological determinants of poor health, and the economic, psychological, social, and cultural factors that contribute to health and illness—the social determinants of health.
- Care for all patients regardless of their ability to pay, and advocate for the medically underserved.
- Be accountable, both ethically and financially.
- Be thoughtful, compassionate, and collegial.
- Continue to learn, and strive for excellence.
- Work to advance the field of medicine, and share knowledge for the benefit of others.
- Reflect dispassionately on your actions, behaviors, and decisions to improve knowledge, skills, judgment, decision making, accountability, and professionalism.

These are, without doubt, very high standards for any individual to live up to, and they would have guided Dr. Richmond's professional and personal life. Imagine if politicians or business executives had to live up to similar standards. Outcomes in those areas would be very different, but individuals would be more highly respected. It is not surprising that patients treat physicians with a great deal of respect. Although physicians pay a cost to uphold these standards, most doctors are able to do so and to achieve a reasonable work-life balance that allows them to be proud of their professional capacities.

Let us turn to lawsuits against doctors and the acknowledged major impact that these can have, as was seen with Dr. Richmond, who ended up ceasing his research activities after being sued. Medscape has issued several *Malpractice Reports* on this topic; a recent one (Levy and Kane 2017) described the impact of lawsuits on more than 4,000 physicians from more than 25 specialty areas. Among the respondents, 55% had been named on the suits, about half of them more than once. Both surgeons and obstetrician-gynecologists led the specialties, with 85% of respondents being sued. Of those physicians who had been sued, 87% said that they were surprised at being sued and almost all believed the suit was unwarranted. Most suits were reported to be for failed diagnoses or treatment. One-third of physicians reported spending more than 40 hours of work on their defense, and only 60% were settled within 2 years. The vast majority of cases settled before or at trial, and it is important to note that only 2% of cases actually went to trial, with the jury deciding against the physicians. These cases are expensive, and the Medscape report indicated that 68% of plaintiffs received up to $500,000, with 17% receiving between $500,000 and $1 million. Very importantly, as a consequence of the lawsuits, 26% of physicians sued said that they no longer trusted their patients, and another 6% changed their practice setting, with 33% of those who were sued saying it negatively affected their career.

Levy (2017) focused on the long-term impact of lawsuits on physicians, noting that during a lawsuit, physicians often experience anxiety, anguish, depression, a sense of betrayal, and shame and feel that the emotional distress will last a lifetime. She found that after a lawsuit is settled or resolved, many doctors respond in one of three ways: 1) they may leave or change their practice, as Dr. Richmond did, 2) they may retire early, or 3) they may lose faith in patients and start to see them as potential adversaries for the remainder of their careers. Not surprisingly, for individuals brought up in a professional environment where ethical behavior is so strongly taught and practiced, the effect of being sued by those for whom one is caring is potentially much greater than in non-medical lawsuits. To a certain extent, psychologically, it is the equivalent of a parent being sued by a child—both surprising and distressing. Given that we know a large number of physicians have experienced long-term effects from being sued, it seems obvious that this is one area in which physicians could be helped. Perhaps a lawsuit should be treated as though it were a sentinel event by both physicians and their employers, in which case, a series of supportive and preventive therapeutic approaches could be automatically offered to the physician being sued, as frequently happens in other traumatic situations. A number of health systems are starting to create such expert peer support options as a counterweight to the inevitable advice from lawyers to say nothing to anyone. If Dr. Richmond had had a supportive, trained colleague to talk with about his lawsuit and how best to handle it, he may have not stopped his research, a part of his practice he especially enjoyed that helped maintain his work balance.

Finally, given the pressures on doctors during their careers, why is it that physicians do not look after themselves better from a medical perspective and take the sort of preventive steps, such as being seen regularly by a primary care provider, that they constantly advise their patients to do? Some excellent books have been written on this topic (Figley et al. 2013). It is said that up to 30% of doctors do not have a primary care physician, but this figure is really uncertain and not backed by any solid evidence. What is more, a recent study from the Kaiser Family Foundation (2018) found that 28% of U.S. men and 17% of U.S. women do not have a primary care physician, with numbers being even higher in minority groups, such as Hispanic males, where 47% reported not having a primary care physician. Whatever the actual figures for doctors, it seems counterintuitive that physicians would not routinely have their own primary care physicians, but it is a fact. We know that physicians, as students and onward, are trained to ignore their own physical and emotional well-being and often keep these habits lifelong. The medical student who has just completed a 24-hour shift feels a sense of pride, even though, by the end of it, he or she is too tired to be safe. Many physicians literally treat themselves and their families for all illnesses, whereas others use denial, a psychological defense common among clinicians, and just assume bad things will not happen to them. Other physicians do not visit colleagues because they are not convinced of those colleagues' competency or, in the case of depression and burnout, because of the stigma associated with mental health. Finally, physicians are taught to be highly self-reliant and resilient, and the unintended consequence of that can be that they do not trust other doctors or do not believe those doctors are as medically good as themselves. It is probably this combination of denial and arrogance that led to Dr. Richmond ignoring the advice of his cardiologist colleague and continuing to work, despite his angina, without getting himself fully assessed and treated.

This first chapter is intended to set the scene for the book by examining the medical environment and the culture of physicians in contrast with family perspectives and some of the unintended consequences. Dr. Richmond is very typical of many hard-working, resilient physicians who continue to exist today and who are highly professional and very caring and concerned for their patients. Many families accept the physician's lifestyle, which puts patients first and often involves not only long hours at work but also long hours of work at home. What will be interesting to see is whether this stereotypical model of a successful physician continues to exist to the same extent in future years. Although Baby-Boomer physicians are likely to continue to maintain these hardworking lifestyles, it is hard to envisage the same choices being made by a high proportion of the Millennial or Generation X physicians of the future who are today's students and residents. They likely will learn from today's physicians, as illustrated in this chapter, and perhaps develop differently and with more focus on work-life balance.

A metaphor I use to illustrate the set of changes required is to start thinking of the physician of today as though he or she were a professional athlete. Both groups have a long, arduous, and expensive training that involves much personal sacrifice for a perceived major goal, and both have to perform at their peak, often frequently and for long periods of time, for which they receive generous financial reward. However, only one group tends to receive substantial physical and psychological support if they are unable to perform at their best, is routinely given rest and time off to recharge, is able to sleep uninterrupted and work reasonable hours, has a fan base that publicizes their successes (and their failures), and can rapidly become a respected celebrity well known locally and nationally. We need to think of physicians as being more like professional athletes, and this is discussed throughout this book.

References

ABIM Foundation, ACP-ASIM Foundation, European Federation of Internal Medicine: Medical professionalism in the new millennium: a physician charter. Ann Intern Med 136:243–246, 2002 11827500

Anzia J: Culture, strategies and the long game: changing the way we prepare medical students and residents for rewarding lives in medicine. Presented at the American College of Psychiatrists, Honolulu, HI, February 21, 2019

Byyny RL, Paauw DS, Papadakis M, et al: Medical Professionalism Best Practices: Professionalism in the Modern Era. Aurora, CO, Alpha Omega Alpha Honor Medical Society, 2017. Available at: http://alphaomegaalpha.org/pdfs/Monograph2018.pdf. Accessed June 8, 2018.

Elton C: Also Human: The Inner Lives of Doctors. New York, Basic Books, 2018

Figley C, Huggard P, Rees CE: First Do No Self-Harm: Understanding and Promoting Physician Stress Resilience. New York, Oxford University Press, 2013

Gabbard GO: The role of compulsiveness in the normal physician. JAMA 254(20):2926–2929, 1985 4057513

Health Professions Advising: Hippocratic Oath, modern version, in UC Davis 2018 Student Handbook. Sacramento, University of California, Davis, 2018. Available at: https://hpa.ucdavis.edu/sites/g/files/dgvnsk4121/files/inline-files/2018Pre-MedBootcampWorkbook.pdf. Accessed September 14, 2019.

Kaiser Family Foundation: Percent of men who report having no personal doctor/health care provider, by race/ethnicity. State Health Facts (website). San Francisco, CA, Kaiser Family Foundation, 2018. Available at: https://www.kff.org/disparities-policy/state-indicator/percent-of-men-who-report-having-no-personal-doctorhealth-care-provider-by-raceethnicity. Accessed June 6, 2018.

Kay A: This Is Going to Hurt: Secret Diaries of a Junior Doctor. New York, Pan Macmillan Australia/Picador, 2017

Levy S: Physicians react: life after a lawsuit. Medscape (website), June 14, 2017. Available at: https://www.medscape.com/viewarticle/880269. Accessed June 12, 2018.

Levy S, Kane L: Medscape malpractice report 2017. MedScape (website), November 15, 2017. Available at: https://www.medscape.com/slideshow/2017-malpractice-report-6009206. Accessed June 11, 2018.

National Academy of Medicine: Action Collaborative on Clinician Well-Being and Resilience Knowledge Hub (website). Washington, DC, National Academy of Medicine, 2019. Available at: https://nam.edu/initiatives/clinician-resilience-and-well-being. Accessed April 3, 2019.

NEJM Catalyst: Physician burnout: the root of the problem and the path to solutions. NEJM Catalyst, June 2018. Available at: https://www.catalyst.nejm.org/download/physician-burnout-collection. Accessed April 3, 2019.

Royal College of Physicians and Surgeons of Canada: The CanMeds Project. Ottawa, ON, Royal College of Physicians and Surgeons of Canada, 2016. Available at: http://www.royalcollege.ca/rcsite/canmeds/framework/canmeds-role-professional-e. Accessed September 21, 2019.

Tanenbaum S: 25 most memorable TV doctors. Everyday Health (website), August 2011. Available at: https://www.everydayhealth.com/healthy-living-pictures/25-most-memorable-tv-doctors.aspx. Accessed June 8, 2018.

Yellowlees P: Physician Suicide: Cases and Commentaries. Washington, DC, American Psychiatric Association Publishing, 2018

Chapter 2

HEALTH CARE IS A TEAM SPORT

Scenario

Health Care Blog, 6 Months Ago

Dear readers,

We are following up on the longstanding rumors about severe dissatisfaction, high burnout, and excessive turnover levels among physicians at University City Health (UCH) in Washington State. Finally, the state's patient complaints unit has gone public with descriptions of poor-quality care and a number of pending lawsuits, as well as low morale among the nursing staff, that culminated with a very poor performance at a recent Joint Commission inspection. Although the results of the inspection are not yet formalized, feedback given to the UCH leadership team indicated that several major citations would be issued and extensive changes needed. It is rumored that the board is unhappy with several C-suite incumbents and may be taking action soon to replace some of these. Our understanding is that these changes will likely include at least the chief executive officer (CEO) and chief medical officer (CMO) being asked to leave. We have tried to get comments from UCH, with no success. The hospital has, however, confirmed our report last week that the nationally known UCH microvascular surgery program has been closed following its loss of accreditation for training residents, two major lawsuits, and the departure of three out of four main vascular surgeons. The situation at UCH is clearly very fluid, and we will continue to report on this.

Health Care Blog, 3 Months Ago

Dear readers,

Once again, this week we focus on the troubles at UCH. Until a few years ago, UCH was nationally recognized as a leader in inpatient care, especially in the surgical area, but now it is seemingly heading in a downward spiral toward a very uncertain future. As we reported previously, CEO Bill Jameston was fired following the dreadful Joint Commission survey, amid a slate of wider accusations of poor personnel management and nepotism involving the employment of several family members. The UCH physicians group appears to be battling internally with the leadership over what they believe has been poor resource allocation and a leadership focus on financial management over clinical care. We understand another four senior physicians have resigned in the past month and that the emergency medicine residency program may well lose its accreditation soon. The only bright spot for UCH seems to be the rapid appointment of Brian Gordon, M.D., as interim CEO. Dr. Gordon was drafted into the position via an agreement with the California UCH Hospital Group, where he has a stellar reputation, and was able to transfer rapidly to Washington State to take up the interim position for reportedly at least 1 year. Dr. Gordon is becoming somewhat of a turnaround expert, having been placed in two troubled hospitals previously, both of which he resurrected by bringing in an almost entirely new management team. We wait with anticipation to see what he does at UCH.

University City Health Administrative Offices, 1 Month Ago

Dr. Gordon, the recently appointed CEO of UCH, shook Dr. Sierra's hand and showed her to a chair. "Thank you for attending this interview, Dr. Sierra. We really appreciate your interest in the position of CMO at University City Health. I know that you have already spent considerable time with the search firm and have had the opportunity to learn about us, just as we have learned about you. We hope this interview will be helpful for all of us and will give you the opportunity to ask further questions about the position. Before we get started, let's go around the table and introduce ourselves."

Dr. Sierra, a well-dressed woman in her forties, sat and listened carefully. Although the interview had not begun in earnest, she felt confident and knew she was making a good first impression on the committee. She smiled at Dr. Gordon and then carefully focused on the whole committee, five men and two women, sitting around the highly polished maple boardroom table. Dr. Sierra knew their backgrounds from her research on the UCH leadership, so as they introduced themselves, she mentally reviewed her plan for starting the interview. She had to be careful not to offend or appear disrespectful to the group. She assumed several of them were likely responsible, at least in part, for the well-publicized problems in the media and the courts that had beset UCH over the past 5 years, and that if she were successful in this job interview, some of them likely would not be retained. She thought about their roles and what she knew about them.

The chief of staff, Dr. Stone, on her immediate left, was a serious-looking, relatively young female anesthesiologist wearing her green scrubs under a lab coat. She wore little makeup, and her light brown hair was tied back. She had just been elected to this role by the UCH medical staff, and Dr. Sierra knew from her research that Dr. Stone was internally quite powerful and on a fast track to administrative promotion. Dr. Stone had been quoted frequently in the media and had led the medical staff in their publicly reported fights against the prior administration. She was quite a contrast to her predecessor, Dr. Rogers, who was seated next to her. He had appeared in the press as a frail, elderly surgeon who frequently seemed to be caught wearing wrinkled scrubs and an exhausted look. Next to him sat Dr. Riley, the director of quality, an ophthalmologist who was nearing retirement and seemed to have little role or influence at UCH. Both physicians sat looking at their interview papers rather than at her. They were quite a contrast to Dr. Gordon, the new CEO, sitting opposite her at the end of the table. He appeared friendly and engaged, eyeing her directly. She knew he was a forward-looking, rather driven endocrinologist who had been appointed to this new role after the appalling Joint Commission report and sudden resignation of the prior CEO a year before. One of Dr. Gordon's first actions had been to fire the previous CMO, which had led to this job interview. The final physician on the panel, Dr. Burtone, was the chairperson of the department of pediatrics, a longstanding and seemingly quite successful individual heading one of the few departments that did not have major physician recruitment problems. She wore a lab coat adorned by a large, handwritten badge announcing her as "Doctor Anna."

The other two interviewers were the nonmedical members of the panel. Mr. Carney, the director of patient care services, was another long-term staff member who had been heavily criticized in the press.

The last person was the director of public relations and marketing, Ms. Odono, a new recruit who was quite successfully starting the essential process of rebranding UCH. *Quite a job*, Dr. Sierra thought to herself. In the weeks prior to this interview she had researched all the UCH senior leadership, and having now met her interview panel, it seemed clear that the power and decision-making capacities in this group lay mainly with the CEO and the chief of staff. She decided to focus primarily on them in her responses.

"So, Dr. Sierra, now that we've all been introduced, and given that the members of this committee have read your application and resume, perhaps we can begin. Would you mind telling us why you are interested in this position, and what you plan to do early on if you are appointed?" Dr. Gordon said.

"Thank you, Dr. Gordon, and thanks to all of you here for taking the time to review my application and meet with me." Dr. Sierra looked around the group, pleased to be taking the stage at last. She spoke comfortably to the panel as a group. "I am aware from my background research of some of the difficulties that UCH has had over the past several years, more publicly so in the past year. However, as an outsider, I cannot pretend to really understand the breadth and depth of these difficulties, so please bear this in mind; I expect it will take at least a couple of months, if I am appointed, to really understand the dynamics of what has been happening. So, with that caveat, let me explain why I am here." Dr. Sierra smiled at the group and noted that all were paying full attention to her.

"You know from my background that my main focus in recent years has been on organizational change, and how to do this in a positive manner that improves both patient outcomes and staff and physician morale. As part of my MBA[1] program several years ago, I worked with the team that developed the 'Triple Aim' of better health for the population, better care for individuals, and cheaper costs. This triple aim was taken up widely around the country, including at UCH. In my view, however, this three-legged stool has been superseded by a four-legged chair that includes a fourth leg of clinician wellness."

Dr. Sierra could see Dr. Gordon nodding positively, obviously aware of the important attitudinal change increasingly being adopted by hospitals and health systems around the country. She continued.

---

[1]MBA=Master of Business Administration.

"The first thing, for me, is to ensure that all of you, and your other leadership colleagues, are aware of this important practical issue and that we adopt this quadruple aim at UCH. Why? Well, my research shows that little focus has been paid in the past on clinician well-being, especially that of physicians. This has led not only to poor physician morale, increased levels of burnout and turnover, and worsened patient care but also to poor morale among all other staff who work with your physicians. It is hardly surprising that if the main cog in a machine isn't working properly, then the rest of the machine becomes less functional. Health care is a team sport; if the quarterback is injured, the whole team is adversely affected."

Dr. Sierra wanted to know now where the interview panel stood on this issue; if she could expect no support for this approach, she wanted to know early so she could decide whether to go forward with her application. She decided to find out and turned toward Dr. Gordon.

"Dr. Gordon, I am aware that you have been in your role only for a few months. What do you think of endorsing and promoting the quadruple aim as a way of reinvigorating UCH and putting a real focus on the staff, especially key physicians on whom the entire system depends?"

"Thanks for bringing up this important topic so early in the interview," Dr. Gordon responded. "I am delighted to discuss this and to endorse the approach. My only concern is that if we implement this quadruple aim, we must have solid plans in place to improve the support and morale of our physician group. There's nothing worse than announcing a new approach but having no practical plan for implementing it. What are your ideas on that, Dr. Sierra?"

Dr. Sierra was pleased with this response, but before she could answer, Dr. Stone interrupted. She spoke excitedly.

"It is so good to be listening to this conversation! I know we haven't spoken before, Dr. Sierra, but this is exactly the sort of approach that the medical staff, or at least those of us who are left, have been promoting! I'm so pleased you see wellness as a cornerstone of your plan, and I look forward to what you propose. You mentioned football players; I wonder if you've heard the metaphor about teams in health care that compares physicians with athletes in terms of their training and support needs? It was presented at a conference I attended recently. Both groups share a lot of similarities—they require many years of training, very high performance levels with few or no mistakes, continuous learning and striving for improvement, and appropriate rest and sustenance. This rest has to be physical, psychological, and social, of course, and strong support systems must be in place to help maintain or improve performance when necessary."

Dr. Stone continued, her tone becoming reflective. "Although physicians do get many of their needs fulfilled, they tend to be very bad at asking for help if everything is not going well, so they miss out on extra coaching or the equivalent of sports psychologists when needed. They often work way too many hours with little or no rest, to the detriment of their home and social lives. And whereas athletes ultimately are measured only on whether they win or lose, physicians are measured by numerous groups—patients, colleagues, administrators, multiple data comparisons of outcomes and activity, and an increasing series of bureaucratic reporting requirements. All of these—to my mind—*absurd* reporting necessities put extra pressure on us and take us away from our core goal of providing great patient care, which is why we chose medicine as a career in the first place."

Dr. Stone had been speaking passionately. Realizing that she was taking up too much time, she came to a sudden stop. "I'm sorry to get on my soapbox, Dr. Sierra, but I do wonder what you think about all this."

Dr. Sierra smiled. The conversation was going in the direction she wanted, and she was extremely pleased with the responses of Drs. Gordon and Stone. It seemed she had at least two strong supporters for the approaches she wanted to implement at UCH. She decided to lay out some of her ideas.

"First, please don't apologize, Dr. Stone. I agree with you about the athlete metaphor. I also am very pleased, Dr. Gordon, to hear your endorsement of the quadruple aim approach. Although the CMO position I'm applying for involves much more than supporting physicians and other providers—and I have numerous ideas for improving the administrative systems, especially around quality and credentialing—I think the immediate task we need to focus on at UCH is restoring morale and stopping the exodus of physicians. I'm sure you know that your largest competitor, West Health, has actually drawn up a list of 'target' UCH physicians whom they are trying to recruit."

While other committee members nodded in affirmation, Mr. Carney, the director of patient care services, responded. "Yes, we are aware of that situation, Dr. Sierra, and we have approached them about it, but with little success. Health care is such a cutthroat business; it sometimes feels as though we are a wounded animal surrounded by vultures."

"Sadly, you are right," Dr. Sierra answered. "And if you don't make rapid solid changes, the vultures may well disembowel you. If I am appointed, my first focus will be on the whole area of physician well-being, and I will need considerable support from the leadership team, as well as an appropriate budget, to implement my strategy. Having said that, I believe now is a really good time to do this. It will be a strong message to all current UCH physicians that they are respected and valued, which will, I hope, have a positive impact on morale."

Dr. Stone enthusiastically endorsed what Dr. Sierra was saying. "I'm sure you're right. Such a proposal will be seen as a very positive move by most of our physicians, many of whom have been here for most of their careers and are heavily invested in the academic mission of UCH. Can you give us some broad details of what you would like to do?"

"Certainly. The first component is to communicate what we wish to do and to keep communicating with all of our physicians, especially about UCH formally adopting the quadruple aim as the core of its strategic plan. I would like to create a new leadership position, probably half-time at first, that we will call the chief wellness officer, or CWO, and some sort of advisory board on physician well-being. This CWO position will be filled by an internal candidate; from what Dr. Stone says, it seems several people may be interested. He or she will need two or three analytic and communications staff and, I assume, will adopt the three-domain Stanford Wellness Framework,[2] which involves creating a culture of wellness, improved efficiency of practice, and better personal resilience across UCH and the physician group. We can put some of those parameters into their job description.

"Much of the work of the CWO will depend on regular measurements and results, and I really don't have a good handle on what UCH has done already and whether burnout or well-being have been measured here in the past. Whatever has been done, we will need to put in place some measurement processes over time and also survey the physicians about what they see as major unfilled needs or as obstructions to providing excellent clinical care. Then we have to keep communicating internally and externally, particularly highlighting excellent practices, individuals, and teams. Lots of other options and initiatives can be implemented over time, but to me, the most important aspect of this strategy is to change the culture at UCH so that clinician well-being really does become one of the core legs of the UCH quadruple aim—in fact and action, not just in name."

As she spoke, Dr. Sierra observed the interview panel and was pleased to see positive responses from Drs. Gordon and Stone, although

---

[2]Stanford Medical Center 2019.

the other physicians in the group seemed fairly neutral. Dr. Stone caught her eye and asked the first question.

"Tell me about the 'improved efficiency of practice' part of this strategy. That sounds a bit like more potential pressure on our physicians, at least in the short term, if it involves yet more change. I think many of my colleagues already have what they call 'change toxicity' and are wary of being required to change their practices or clinical workflows again. In the past, such changes usually have been made primarily to increase the revenue base, not necessarily to improve clinical care."

"I understand your colleagues' concerns, Dr. Stone. Any such efficiency changes would have to be undertaken very carefully and with full consultation with all those involved. The aim is to take pressure off physicians, give them more time with patients and have them spend less time on administrative tasks and documentation, especially the EMR.[3] You've probably heard of one recent article that described how to get rid of what was called 'stupid stuff,' defined as anything in the EMR that was badly designed or unnecessary?"

Several people nodded.

"Let me give you one other quick example of potential changes," she continued. "Do you think that American doctors practice medicine very differently from their European counterparts?"

"No," answered Dr. Stone. "I spent a month in Paris as a resident on an elective and was surprised at how similar the quality of medicine was. In fact, in some areas, such as infectious diseases, the French are way ahead of us."

"So, if their practice standards are similar, would you assume that they write approximately the same number of notes per patient?"

Dr. Stone considered the question. "Probably not. I suspect that U.S. doctors actually write somewhat more notes, because we tend to practice more defensively and are more frequently being sued, and we have some ridiculous requirements for billing. So maybe American doctors might write—as a guess—up to twice as much as European doctors? But I'd be surprised if it was really that much extra."

"Well, you would be wrong," replied Dr. Sierra. "A recent comparison of European and American medical notes showed that U.S. doctors actually write between three and five times as much as European doctors, and for no obvious clinical benefit. Can you imagine how much extra time that takes away from patient care, and how much extra 'pajama

---

[3]EMR=electronic medical record.

time' our physicians spend after hours and on weekends working on their notes as a result? It's awful! One of the areas I would look at is excess documentation. For this, it would be necessary to work with both payers and physicians to educate everyone about this issue and start allowing physicians to write less—while still writing good clinical notes. A massive amount of time could be saved here, and not just by the physicians who are writing the notes. I'm sure you've read many notes where patients are seen each month and a long note is often copied and pasted into the record with very few changes. When you see this patient, perhaps for the first time, you have to read through ridiculous volumes of repetitive notes to find comments about changing clinical status. Wouldn't it be so much simpler to have one initial comprehensive note and then multiple follow-up notes that identify only important clinical issues? You could review the notes in half the time and be much less likely to miss important clinical changes. Think of the average wiki and imagine that as a constantly updated patient medical record."

Dr. Gordon looked up from the file in front of him. "Huh. That is really amazing, when you think of it like that. I didn't realize these data were so compelling. Thank you for telling us. The potential time savings would be huge for both the doctors who are writing and those who are reviewing the notes. That would mean more time with patients and likely less burnout and dissatisfaction."

The interview continued for another half an hour, with questions from all members of the panel all expertly fielded by Dr. Sierra. By the end of the agreed time, the atmosphere in the room was friendly and collegial, and the interview had morphed into what appeared to be a friendly discussion among colleagues rather than a high-stakes meeting. Dr. Sierra, however, although inwardly confident about her performance and her qualifications for the CMO position, knew that she had one last enormous fence to jump if she were to be appointed, a fence she had failed to jump several times already in interviews for similar positions. She knew the only way to handle it was head on during the interview.

When Dr. Gordon moved to finish up the interview and asked if she had any further questions or comments to make, she surprised everyone by asking to tell a story about herself for them to consider. She looked around the panel and then deliberately focused on Dr. Stone, whom she believed likely to be most sympathetic. Dr. Sierra started speaking directly to her, trying to follow the advice of her psychiatrist to forget that she was in a high-stakes interview and to imagine she was telling her story to a compassionate colleague in a coffee shop.

"I hope it's clear that I have the academic and professional experience to successfully become your CMO. However, I need to tell you about one issue that you will find in my credentialing papers if you decide to consider appointing me to this position. I would rather tell you about this myself, here at the interview, so you can hear my side of the story directly rather than just assume that the papers and decisions from the medical board are correct and fair. I will be quick with my story, and I thank you for listening to me."

The interview panel, who previously had been winding down and starting to relax at the end of what they all thought was a most impressive interview, suddenly became more alert at this unusual finale. Dr. Gordon, in particular, was mystified and concerned, because he had been particularly impressed by Dr. Sierra and felt confident that he had found a first-class CMO with whom he could work well. He especially liked her interest in physician well-being and her impressive, thoroughly considered strategies to improve physician morale and retention. He watched her and listened intently, with no idea where Dr. Sierra was going with this unusual closing statement.

"I went into medicine because I wanted to help people, and that is still my passion," Dr. Sierra began. "Unfortunately, my family includes several people who have been depressed, including my grandmother, who raised me after my mother died from suicide a month after I was born. My own first bout of depression occurred in medical school, and since then I have had five serious episodes, only one of which led to me taking any time off work when I was a junior attending about 12 years ago. At that time, I was given very bad advice by a senior colleague; I was advised to voluntarily tell the medical board about my depression and that it was why, on the advice of my psychiatrist at the time, I was taking a month off work. Since then, I have been in a battle with the medical board, although I did not employ lawyers until about 7 years ago when they tried to take away my medical license completely. I have never been impaired to practice; have never been psychotic or so ill that I was dangerous to myself or others; have never been certified or admitted to a psychiatric hospital; have never tried to kill myself; and have never had a drug or alcohol problem. I have sought help and have a regular psychiatrist and psychotherapist, and I take long-term medications that have helped me greatly. I have not had to take time off work because of depression in the past 12 years."

Dr. Sierra sat back, still looking intently at Dr. Stone but also carefully scanning the rest of the interview panel for their reaction. Would they suddenly think of her very differently? She decided to continue her story without giving them a chance to interrupt.

"What I have discovered, however, is a horrendous level of bias and stigma against doctors who are labeled as mentally ill, and how this pervades the licensing system and some of the staff that they employ, as well as other hospital credentialing groups. Immediately after I shared my story with the board, I was forced to stop practicing for 3 months until I could prove to one of the medical board investigators, a nonclinician, that I was fit to work again—despite my own psychiatrist giving me a return-to-work fitness note after 4 weeks. I was required to go into a supervised practice program and to do random alcohol and drug tests for 3 years, despite never having had such a problem, because apparently they considered me at risk for self-medicating with alcohol because of my depression. If you look at my license on the medical board website, it will say that it is unrestricted, now that I have gotten lawyers involved, but it also shows a long history of licensing restrictions that I cannot get removed and that are there for anyone to read. My whole professional life has been turned upside down by this situation, and I have been turned down for a number of jobs as a result, despite my excellent qualifications and references."

Dr. Stone looked very compassionately toward Dr. Sierra, clearly touched by this story. She was aware of how difficult it must have been for Dr. Sierra to bring it up at the interview and to be so open about her situation. She knew several of her colleagues were likely to treat this background information as a fatal flaw, and she wanted to give Dr. Sierra the opportunity to present herself as well as possible.

"I really appreciate you being so direct about this situation, Dr. Sierra," she said. "It cannot be easy to address such a personal issue, and one with such unfortunate and apparently long-term professional consequences. Thank you. I wonder if you could confirm with us, as you have brought it up at the interview, what your health status currently is, and whether you have any outstanding licensing or credentialing issues that we need to know about."

"Thank you, Dr. Stone. I appreciate your kind comments. This is not an easy situation for me, nor for you, I am sure. I've learned that it's best to be completely up front about my past rather than wait for you to discover it when you run my background check, if you decide I am a potentially appointable candidate. I would rather be completely honest from the beginning of any professional relationship, and I am particularly keen to be appointed to UCH, because I see so much that is positive here. My psychiatrist, whom I have seen for about 8 years now, tells me she thinks I am so enthused about this job because of some unconscious parallels I am drawing between UCH and myself, but I'm not sure about that. She thinks I want to help turn UCH around, just as I have turned myself around, because she knows there are many excellent physicians at UCH who have done nothing wrong, just as I did nothing wrong by reporting my illness to the medical board. Anyway, whatever the case, what I can do is assure you that I now have a full, unrestricted medical license after 7 years of legal fighting and considerable expense.

"I also know that I have a diagnosis of recurrent major depressive disorder with a likely strong genetic component and that I am well and have a strong therapeutic team in place to help me with any future relapses. As a result, I should neither need to take time off work nor have any level of medical impairment. I have no other medical illnesses, and my depressive disorder has overall caused me to have much less disability or loss of work time than if I had diabetes, arthritis, or cardiac problems. I'm not sure if you have any questions you would like to put to me now, but I welcome these if you have. Whatever your reaction to my story, I hope you will bear what I have said in mind as you make your decisions and if you feel you need to review the various documents about me on the medical board website."

Dr. Sierra sat back, satisfied that she had given a reasonable description of her difficulties and pleased that she had remained objective and had not been excessively defensive in her self-description. She flicked her head sideways, brushed aside some stray hairs that had fallen over her left eye, and surveyed the room. She was uncertain as to the panel's response, although she noted sympathetic smiles from several members. She turned toward Dr. Gordon and waited for his comments, because she knew that her time with the panel was now well over. He thanked her for her honesty and preparedness to openly discuss an obviously very painful but important sequence of events. After receiving his additional thanks for attending the interview, Dr. Sierra left the room.

Dr. Gordon turned to his colleagues and initiated an immediate discussion about her. "I would like to hear what you all thought of Dr. Sierra, and whether you think she is appointable as our CMO. As you all know, she was our top choice on paper and has considerably more experience than any of the other candidates we have reviewed. Like all of you, I suspect, I was not aware of her past licensing situation or of her longstanding mental illness, and I think we certainly have to take those issues into account as we make our decision about whether to appoint her. I seek all of your opinions and expect that they will inform mine. Who would like to go first?"

Rather to Dr. Gordon's surprise, the first three speakers were the surgeon, the ophthalmologist, and the director of patient care services, who between them had contributed least to the interview so far. They all spoke positively about Dr. Sierra's qualifications overall but made it clear they thought that appointing her would be too great a risk for UCH. Their concerns were broadly twofold. First, they thought that UCH would be further criticized in the press if it became widely known that the new CMO had had a lot of medical licensing problems, and that these problems might impair her relationship with the medical board. They argued that this could be a challenge in her role as CMO, where she was inevitably going to have regular interactions with the board about other UCH doctors and would need to have a good working relationship with them. Second, they were concerned that she had what they described as a chronic mental illness, which they felt might impair her judgment in the future and made her unfit, in their opinion, to hold a C-suite position.

Dr. Gordon listened patiently to all three and deliberately asked the director of marketing, Julie Odono, for her comments next. Dr. Gordon had come to rely on Ms. Odono for her rapid and accurate assessments of individuals whom she met and for her direct and honest feedback to him if she thought he was making an error in judgment. She did not surprise him when she immediately took a very different view from the previous speakers.

"I have to say that I totally disagree with what the others have been saying. I thought she was superb, and I would love to work with her. From my perspective in marketing, she is someone whom I believe will represent UCH excellently, and I cannot wait to get her in front of the media. She will be able to defend herself, I'm sure. Having said that, we obviously have to do some due diligence about her licensing issues and review what has occurred, but I believe her. I've seen other physicians run into similar problems with medical boards, and also with some physician health programs, and I'm sure that if you Googled it, you would find quite a few similar anecdotal experiences. I'm not trying to be critical of medical boards, who have a hard job, but their primary purpose is to protect the consumer, not the doctor. Undoubtedly, in some situations they have to make decisions based on their requirements that can place undue burdens on physicians from our perspective. I would be happy to help investigate this situation, and that may even involve further discussions with Dr. Sierra herself. Let's not rush to judgment on the licensing issue. I give her kudos for bringing it up herself in such an important interview.

"On the issue of her having a mental illness, I am just surprised that you three intelligent health professionals take the view you do. If we were to ban all people with such disorders from C-suites around the country, we would lose many of our best business and health leaders. These illnesses are very common, and as a health system we should take the lead and never discriminate against those who have them, as long as they are not impaired. And no evidence that she has ever been impaired has been reported, from what I heard."

Dr. Burtone, the chief of pediatrics, spoke next in her usual careful, measured tone.

"I have to say that I agree with Julie completely. I thought Dr. Sierra was a breath of fresh air, and someone whom we really need. I liked her personally and would feel very comfortable reporting to her, and I believe my other chair colleagues will as well. I thought she had a very strong side to her, almost steely, especially in the way that she has overcome obstacles. To have completed her MBA and to have such stellar references at a time when she was fighting for her professional life with the medical board and getting a handle on her own depression is simply amazing. I agree that we have to do our due diligence about the licensing issue, but I think she is just the sort of person to help lead UCH out of its dreadful mess. And from what I understand, her husband is also an excellent surgeon; if we get her, we might also recruit him, which is an excellent add-on bonus—although I know we are not meant to take note of such situations during her recruitment."

"Thanks indeed, Dr. Burtone. I really appreciate your comments. You're right; if we can recruit her, we may also be recruiting part of a real power couple who could help draw other talent to UCH," said Dr. Gordon. "Over to you, Dr. Stone, although I suspect I know in which direction you are likely to move."

"I think you do, Dr. Gordon. I must have made my attitude toward Dr. Sierra fairly obvious during the interview. Clearly, I agree with Julie and Anna, and I would welcome Dr. Sierra with open arms, assuming that our review of her licensing situation comes out okay. I think she has a very strong professional and administrative background and a good clinical reputation, and she has even written a number of interesting papers on the topic of physician well-being, on which she seems to be quite an expert. We now know part of her motivation for that interest, but it is an interest that suits UCH perfectly, and I really liked her strategic ideas for how to improve our physician morale and efficiency of practice. I thought it was very gutsy of her to bring up this issue so overtly in this interview, even before we have gone down the path of checking her credentials. Others would have waited to find out if they were a preferred candidate and only then would have revealed their background, so she certainly took a risk by being so open with us. But I like that! We need someone who is confident enough to take a risk on themselves. I would totally support her appointment and would be happy to recommend this to the medical staff executive committee if you wish."

"Thanks indeed, Dr. Stone. I like the way you think, and your openness about her," said Dr. Gordon. "It seems that we have two sets of strongly held views about Dr. Sierra, and I appreciate all of you giving me your honest opinions." He paused and looked around the panel, seemingly asserting himself and coming to a conclusion. "When I am selecting someone who will be reporting directly to me, I have long believed that one factor is of greater importance than all others, assuming that the individual is qualified for the position, as Dr. Sierra certainly is. That factor is trust. Do I trust the individual? Will they, to use a political phrase, speak truth to power, and will they always be dependable and someone on whom I can rely? In Dr. Sierra, I think we have found just such a person, and I think she showed us that side of herself today in an unusually brave, and—to use Dr. Stone's word—*gutsy* performance. So, although I will arrange for her licensing situation to be checked out, I do hope you will all support her being offered the position and will keep the conversation we've had with her this afternoon completely confidential. The confidentiality is for both her sake and ours. Thanks to all of you for putting in so much time and effort on this search. I will follow up with Dr. Sierra and see what we can negotiate with her. I have a good feeling about this and really hope we can add her to our team."

Health Care Blog, Present Day

Dear readers,

Is UCH continuing to stumble? Readers will recall the massive problems the hospital has had over the past year with its physicians and the drain of their physician talent to other health systems. Well, UCH has just announced the appointment of Dr. Roseanne Sierra as its new chief medical officer. Dr. Sierra has an excellent academic and business background, so why do I ask if UCH is stumbling again? Well, I suggest you look at Dr. Sierra's background on the medical board website. She was put on probation many years ago after a self-reported psychiatric illness and has been engaged in litigation for several years to clear her name and obtain an unrestricted medical license. Is this really the sort of doctor UCH should be employing to lead its physician practice group? The CEO of UCH, Dr. Gordon, strongly defended Dr. Sierra when asked about her background and said that he looked forward to working with her and did not consider her past history of depression a significant concern. He said that he admired her strength in successfully fighting the medical board to clear her name, and he predicted that she would show similar leadership qualities in her work with UCH. We hope he is right, dear reader, and will be following up closely as she begins her work next month. UCH cannot afford any more stumbles!

Commentary

This story raises two important issues, both of which are increasingly being resolved or reduced through the implementation of a number of changes and solutions.

First is the need for organizational and systemic changes to reduce physician burnout. One strategy is for clinician well-being to become a central leg of any health system or clinic strategic plan, especially in a system like UCH, where physician burnout is prevalent and dysfunction is obvious. The solution for this will likely be through the commitment of leadership, such as Dr. Sierra, and the appointment of a *chief wellness officer* who is empowered to be influential in changing culture, increasing efficiency across the system, and improving self-care broadly. Such strategic changes in an environment like the one described here would be many and substantial and include improvements in wide-ranging areas from childcare access and physician morale to reducing the amount of documentation required in the EMR. The role of a CWO is still relatively new in the United States, and examples of the aims and function of such roles are described herein.

The second major issue for discussion is the importance and widespread occurrence of stigma in relation to psychiatric disorders, especially among health professionals, and the traditional roles of medical boards and licensing authorities in making this stigma worse. Many widely available examples on the internet of individual cases cause significant fear and concern among the physician community. Fortunately, positive changes are coming that should reduce the stigma of mental health disorders and lead medical boards and similar licensing or administrative bodies to focus more on levels of impairment when assessing physicians' capacity for practice than on specific diseases such as addictions or psychiatric illness.

I reviewed the topic of burnout and its development extensively in my book *Physician Suicide: Cases and Commentaries* (Yellowlees 2018), and a lengthy and detailed *NEJM Catalyst* (2018) monograph on the topic is also available. Numerous articles on the diagnosis, prevalence, measuring instruments, and causes of burnout are available in the literature, many coming from the research teams at the Mayo Clinic and Stanford University led by Dr. Lotte Dyrbye and Dr. Tait Shanafelt, respectively (Dyrbye et al. 2017; Shanafelt et al. 2015, 2019a, 2019b; Trockel et al. 2018). A recent systematic review by Panagioti et al. (2018) examined the association between physician burnout and patient safety, physician professionalism, and patient satisfaction. Briefly, the full syndrome of *burnout* is now more specifically defined as consisting of a syndrome of all three of the following symptoms, although most people affected have varying components of these symptoms at any one time:

- *Emotional depletion*—The individual feels emotionally depleted, tired of going to work, and frustrated and finds it hard to deal with other people in the workplace.
- *Detachment and cynicism*—The person is less empathic with patients and feels detached from his or her work, seeing and treating patients as objects or diagnoses rather than humans and primarily as sources of frustration to be dealt with in whatever way is possible.
- *Low personal achievement*—The individual experiences work as unrewarding and feels as though it is not meaningful and that he or she is just going through the motions.

Interestingly, the next version of the *International Classification of Diseases* (ICD-11) will include burnout as a specific medical diagnosis, following a proposal for such a move by the World Health Organization (2019).

Let's focus first on the strategic and organizational changes and solutions to burnout. Dr. Sierra mentioned the Quadruple Aim in her interview. This begs the question of what is the Triple Aim, and why should we be thinking of moving strategically toward a quadruple aim for health care? The best definition of the Triple Aim I have found is on the website of the Institute for Healthcare Improvement (2019), which originated the concept in 2006. Here the definition as applied to populations of patients is "applying integrated approaches to simultaneously improve care, improve population health, and reduce costs per capita."

Over the past decade, there has been a growing understanding that successful health care systems are those that can simultaneously deliver excellent quality of care for individual patients at optimized, reduced costs per person while improving the overall health of their population using various preventive and public health approaches. Most major health systems have adopted the framework of the Triple Aim and have used it to make their care systems as focused on patients as possible. However, in recent years, several organizations have added a fourth aim to the original triple aim strategy. For many organizations, the fourth aim is attaining joy in work, or clinician well-being, as Dr. Sierra suggests in the scenario. For other health systems, it may be pursuing health equity or highlighting other priorities, such as in the military health system, for example, where "readiness" has been added as the fourth aim. Whatever this fourth aim may be, it is important not to stray from the original core component of patient centeredness, as described in the Triple Aim. Many health systems are now moving toward a fourth aim of clinician well-being, recognizing that clinicians have not been prioritized sufficiently in the past and that this must change, and are including this aim in their strategic planning exercises.

What are the potential advantages of moving toward a fourth aim of clinician well-being? This typically occurs in response to what is increasingly being described as an epidemic of burnout, as discussed in my previous book (Yellowlees 2018), where the history and development of the syndrome is fully described. The first and most important advantage relates to culture change and the widespread acknowledgment that a major outcome such as clinician well-being, that is measurable and can be monitored, is essential for any health system. This cultural shift can be incorporated at all levels of staff, and increasingly, metrics measuring it are being included in the position requirements of leaders in major health systems. Many metrics are available, not just burnout surveys, for example, but also staff turnover, absenteeism, patient and staff complaints, and adverse incidents, all of which are indicators or potential results of provider well-being.

Numerous papers and reports now describe the strategic organizational and systemic changes that can be made to improve physician well-being and reduce burnout (Dyrbye et al. 2017). Some are discussed in my previous book (Yellowlees 2018). What is becoming clear is the importance and effectiveness of strategies to both prevent and reduce rates of burnout in physicians, as described in excellent systematic reviews of physician burnout and well-being by Rothenberger (2017) and Shanafelt et al. (2015). In a review of the strategies developed through their longstanding use of organizational approaches to reduce burnout at the Mayo Clinic, Shanafelt and Noseworthy (2017) concluded:

> Our experience demonstrates that deliberate, sustained, and comprehensive efforts by the organization to reduce burnout and promote engagement can make a difference. Many effective interventions are relatively inexpensive, and small investments can have a large impact. Leadership and sustained attention from the highest level of the organization are the keys to making progress. (p. 129)

Shanafelt and Noseworthy (2017) defined nine organizational strategies as follows:

- Acknowledge and assess the problem
- Harness the power of leadership
- Develop and implement targeted interventions
- Cultivate community at work
- Use rewards and incentives wisely
- Align values and strengthen culture
- Promote flexibility and work-life integration
- Provide resources to promote resilience and self-care
- Facilitate and fund organizational science

These strategies to create change are similar in their conclusions to the two excellent online modules produced by the American Medical Association (Brooks 2017; Sinsky et al. 2018) on the prevention of burnout in both residents and physicians, which identify systems-level and individual interventions to prevent burnout and achieve the quadruple aim. The other strategic approach to change culture that is being widely quoted and used is the three domains of the WellMD "professional fulfillment model," which comprises creation of the following (quoted from Stanford Medical Center 2019):

1. A culture of wellness: shared values, behaviors, and leadership qualities that prioritize personal and professional growth, community, and compassion for self and others
2. Efficiency of practice: workplace systems, processes, and practices that promote safety, quality, effectiveness, positive patient and colleague interactions, and work-life balance
3. Personal resilience: individual skills, behaviors, and attitudes that contribute to physical, emotional, and professional well-being

The implementation of these approaches and strategies, as Dr. Sierra was advocating at UCH, make it likely that the organization will improve its alignment with its key clinicians, thereby reducing levels of burnout in physicians by at least 10%–15%. It is not surprising that Dr. Sierra was appointed to the position of CMO, because it is clear that the new leadership at UCH understood that this change of strategy was necessary if they were to move away from the traditional approach of most health systems, which still tend to put most of the focus for change back on individual staff and clinical units. To drive these systemic changes, especially as they relate to the EMR and documentation—getting rid of the "stupid stuff" that Dr. Sierra mentioned and as described by Ashton (2018)—many health systems are now appointing CWOs. These roles are diverse and variable, as described by Mahoney (2018), who interviewed several early appointee CWOs to find out their priorities. These priorities comprised benchmarking and finding solutions for burnout, improving the efficiency of the practice environment, encouraging doctors to do the work they find most meaningful, and encouraging leadership training.

As of April 2019, about 30 CWOs had been formally appointed in the United States, although many other leaders hold different position titles but similar roles. I, myself, have such a role, appointed in November 2018, and it is worth examining the primary expectations as defined in the University of California, Davis CWO position description. The summary describes the role well (Kirk 2018):

> Reporting directly to the Chief Medical Officer, this leadership position is the Chief Wellness Officer for UC Davis Health. The incumbent has primary responsibility for managing and directing Medical Staff wellness and well-being programs and initiatives across UCDH. The position will coordinate with other clinical and administrative health professional groups as relevant.
>
> The CWO's main responsibility is to develop a work culture in which physicians have the opportunity to not only show up and perform, but to thrive.
>
> In addition to being a thought leader in the area of physician wellness, the incumbent directly oversees staff in the Office of Physician Wellness in the Division of Clinical Affairs and has responsibility for coordinating wellness programs and relevant culture change initiatives across all UCDH departments and offices.
>
> The major responsibilities include
>
> - Coordinating all strategic planning efforts on Medical Staff wellness, both short-term and multi-year. The CWO translates the vision—that physician wellness is a critical and essential business component of UCDH—into detailed, tangible, and attainable strategic plans.
> - Collaborate with the UCDH leadership to identify, develop, operationalize and implement strategies and initiatives that target improvement in UCDH culture of wellness, efficiency of practice, and personal resilience. Create a culture and encourage an environment that fosters innovation and change. Anticipate emerging trends and develop leading-edge strategies and plans to prepare for them.
> - Work to develop a menu of physician wellness offerings (including organizational change, individual resilience initiatives,

and educational and research outputs) for UCDH and then help manage these programs from concept to execution.

It is evident from this position description that the role is broad and strategic in nature, focused primarily on organizational and systemic change, and precisely the type of role required in the scenario to energize and stimulate needed change at UCH. Ironically, the major obstruction to this approach in the scenario was whether Dr. Sierra could be appointed to the CMO position. Some members of the appointments committee and the wider community, perhaps also informed by the health care blog, would have to overcome their personal level of stigma associated with psychiatric disorders to make this happen and to ensure that she could retain her position and respect while assisting Dr. Gordon in his endeavors.

Dr. Sierra's story of licensing problems is based broadly on several well-publicized stories of physicians who have had long fights with state medical boards to maintain their license. A tragic recent example is the 10-year-long saga of Dr. Susan Haney (2018), who described her experiences of prejudice, bias, and discrimination, as well as a loss of autonomy and privacy, in great detail. She experienced the presumption by medical licensing boards that her psychiatric diagnosis made her unfit to practice, even though she was not apparently impaired and had self-reported her diagnosis. She spent more than $150,000 in legal fees and ended her fight with an unrestricted medical license but without a "clean record" on the medical board website. She quoted a number of other colleagues who had similar experiences and made the important point that impairment, not diagnosis, is the important factor in determining whether physicians are fit to practice.

Physicians' fear of reporting psychiatric or addiction diagnoses to medical boards is very real, but some boards at least are starting to change. To use California as an example, although most medical boards have similar variations of these questions, when any physician used to apply for a license to the Medical Board of California, among a wide range of other questions about their education and training, they had to answer the following six questions (quoted from Medical Board of California 2018, p. 5):

1. Have you ever been enrolled in, required to enter into, or participated in any drug, alcohol, or substance abuse recovery program or impaired practitioner program?
2. Have you ever been treated for or had recurrence of a diagnosed addictive disorder?

3. Have you ever been diagnosed with an emotional, mental, or behavioral disorder that may impair your ability to practice medicine safely?
4. Have you ever been diagnosed with a neurological or other physical condition that may impair your ability to practice medicine safely?
5. Do you have any other condition that may in any way impair or limit your ability to practice medicine safely?
6. Do you suffer from a progressive disorder or a health condition that will likely result in a general decline in health or function that may impair or limit your ability to practice medicine safely?

All of these questions were very broad and used to strike fear into the hearts of many physicians. Medical students have long been warned about them. All applicants for a medical license know that honesty in all transactions with medical boards is of paramount importance, but they also hear of cases in which reporting minor past psychiatric disorders, such as an episode of depression, led to long investigations and sanctions on licenses. Of course, most people assume that they mainly apply to psychiatric disorders, but what about the surgeon who broke a wrist 5 years previously and was impaired and unable to work— should that be reported as well? What these questions did, sadly, was contribute to the culture of stigma and fear around psychiatric disorders, making physicians literally afraid to seek treatment in the belief that they would have to report such treatment. A physician with a history of well-treated depression who had to take 2 weeks off work at the height of his or her illness used to have to report this and risk potential sanctions, even if the physician had never been impaired or worked while impaired. Consequently, many physicians have for years decided not to make such a report for fear of an inquisition into their mental health. The problem with this situation, apart from the distress caused to the doctors and their families, is that an untreated doctor with, for example, depression or substance abuse, is likely to make more patient errors than a treated doctor, so the ultimate unintended consequence of the intrusive application questions has been, for many years, an increase in morbidity among physicians and worse overall patient care.

Fortunately, the tide is turning on this issue, partly as a consequence of numerous brave physicians making their stories public. A report from the Federation of Medical Boards in April 2018 recommended that state medical boards ask questions focusing on current impairment, and not on illness, diagnosis, or previous treatment, in order to ensure compliance with the Americans with Disabilities Act. As of June 2019, more than 30 medical boards have voted to change their licensing questions. California is one of those that has moved, in May 2019, to only three questions on the license application form focusing on physical or psychological impairment at the time of application (Medical Board of California 2019). The new questions are as follows:

1. Are you currently enrolled in or participating in any drug, alcohol, or substance abuse recovery program or impaired practitioner program?
2. Do you currently have any condition (including, but not limited to emotional, mental, neurological, or other physical addictive or behavioral disorder) that impairs your ability to practice medicine safely?
3. Do you currently have any other condition that impairs or limits your ability to practice medicine safely?

Whatever positive changes happen about the licensing issues, unfortunately, the stigma of mental illness will remain and needs to be constantly addressed as part of the professional cultural change discussed in Chapter 1. Myers (2017, 2018) has described how stigma kills doctors, estimating that 10%–15% of doctors who take their lives have received no treatment for the illness that led them to suicide. He described two types of stigma, both of which are demonstrated in the scenario. *Enacted stigma* is exterior and involves discrimination and prejudice on the implicit belief set that people with psychiatric disorders are inferior or less capable. The blog writer and several of Dr. Sierra's interviewers clearly demonstrated this. For physicians, however, the other type of stigma, *felt stigma*, which is internal, is often worse. This involves the fear of enacted stigma from others and the feeling of shame associated with having a psychiatric illness. This form of stigma was exhibited by Dr. Sierra during her interview, even as she assertively told her story to the panel. She was well aware of how she would be judged and how it would be harder for her to gain the professional trust and respect of her colleagues in her new position.

What are the solutions for the pernicious effect of the stigma of mental illness within the medical profession, and more broadly? Stair (2017) has called for more openness; less hiding and struggling alone; the development of more support and social networks, perhaps via a physician lounge at work or a set of social group activities within the wider community, as described later in Chapter 10; and more sharing of stories and letting others know that they are not alone. The American Medical Association has recognized this problem and views easy access to mental health care as an essential component of the medical school of the future. Psychiatrists and other mental health professionals need to change their attitudes, promote their skills and knowledge across the broader health care system, and continue to integrate their practice into general health care practices while also taking up leadership positions such as CWOs where they can work on the challenge of reducing stigma within the culture of medicine.

Stories designed to reduce the stigma of mental illness and addictions in physicians are increasingly being published in prestigious journals, blogs, and newspapers. The article by Hill (2017) in the *New England Journal of Medicine* is a good example of a self-revelatory description of addiction, depression, and recovery that finishes with some solutions that Dr. Sierra would find helpful. Hill noted:

> Instead of stigmatizing physicians who have sought treatment, we need to break down the barriers we've erected.… Empathy, unity, and understanding can help us shift the cultural framework towards acceptance and support. Mentally healthy physicians are safe, productive, effective physicians. The last lesson is about building a support network. My network has been the bedrock of my recovery. You can start small and gradually add trusted people, from your spouse and family to friends, counselors, support groups, and eventually colleagues. Then when you fall flat on your face, there will be someone to pick you up, dust you off, and say, "Get back out there and try it again." A support network can also hold you accountable, ensuring that you remain true to your own personal and professional standards.

References

Ashton M: Getting rid of stupid stuff. N Engl J Med 379(19):1789–1791, 2018 30403948

Brooks E: Preventing Physician Distress and Suicide. AMA Steps Forward (website). Chicago, IL, American Medical Association, 2017. Available at: https://www.stepsforward.org/modules/preventing-physician-suicide. Accessed April 4, 2019.

Dyrbye LN, Shanafelt TD, Sinsky CA, et al: Burnout Among Health Care Professionals: A Call to Explore and Address this Underrecognized Threat to Safe, High-Quality Care (Discussion Paper). Washington, DC, National Academy of Medicine, July 5, 2017. Available at: https://nam.edu/burnout-among-health-care-professionals-a-call-to-explore-and-address-this-under-recognized- threat-to-safe-high-quality-care. Accessed April 4, 2019.

Haney ST: Emergency physician with depression chronicles her 10-year fight to keep her license. ACEP Now, December 17, 2018. Available at: https://www.acepnow.com/article/emergency-physician-with-depression-chronicles-her-10-year-fight-to-keep-her-license. Accessed April 5, 2019.

Hill AB: Breaking the stigma: a physician's perspective on self-care and recovery. N Engl J Med 376(12):1103–1105, 2017 28328327

Institute for Healthcare Improvement: Triple Aim for Populations (website). Boston, MA, Institute for Healthcare Improvement, 2019. Available at: http://www.ihi.org/Topics/TripleAim/Pages/Overview.aspx. Accessed September 15, 2019.

Kirk JD: Chief Wellness Officer Position Description. Sacramento, CA, Division of Clinical Affairs, UC Davis Health, November 2018

Mahoney S: Doctors in distress. AAMC News, September 4, 2018. Available at: https://news.aamc.org/patient-care/article/doctors-distress. Accessed April 5, 2019.

Medical Board of California: Medical Board of California Licensing Program Application. CA.gov (website), 2018. Available at: http://www.mbc.ca.gov/Forms/Applicants/application_forms_l1a-l1f.pdf. Accessed April 5, 2019.

Medical Board of California: Quarterly Board Meeting Agenda, May 9–10, 2019. Available at: http://www.mbc.ca.gov/Licensees. Accessed September 15, 2019.

Myers MF: Why Physicians Die by Suicide: Lessons Learned From Their Families and Others Who Cared. New York, Michael F. Myers, MD, 2017

Myers MF: How stigma kills doctors. Psychology Today, January 9, 2018. Available at: http://www.mbc.ca.gov/About_Us/Meetings/Agendas/678/brd-Agenda-20190509.pdf. Accessed April 5, 2019.

NEJM Catalyst: Physician burnout: the root of the problem and the path to solutions. NEJM Catalyst, June 2018. Available at: https://www.catalyst.nejm.org/download/physician-burnout-collection. Accessed April 3, 2019.

Panagioti M, Geraghty K, Johnson J, et al: Association between physician burnout and patient safety, professionalism, and patient satisfaction: a systematic review and meta-analysis. JAMA Intern Med 178(10):1317–1330, 2018 30193239

Rothenberger DA: Physician burnout and well-being: a systematic review and framework for action. Dis Colon Rectum 60(6):567–576, 2017 28481850

Shanafelt TD, Noseworthy JH: Executive leadership and physician well-being: nine organizational strategies to promote engagement and reduce burnout. Mayo Clin Proc 92(1):129–146, 2017 27871627

Shanafelt TD, Hasan O, Dyrbye LN, et al: Changes in burnout and satisfaction with work-life balance in physicians and the general US working population between 2011 and 2014. Mayo Clin Proc 90(12):1600–1613, 2015 26653297

Shanafelt TD, Trockel M, Ripp J, et al: Building a program on well-being: key design considerations to meet the unique needs of each organization. Acad Med 94(2):156–161, 2019a 30134268

Shanafelt TD, West CP, Sinsky C, et al: Changes in burnout and satisfaction with work-life integration in physicians and the general US working population between 2011 and 2017. Mayo Clin Proc 2019b 30803733 Epub ahead of print

Sinsky C, Shanafelt TD, Murphy ML, et al: Creating the Organizational Foundation for Joy in Medicine. AMA Steps Forward (website). Chicago, IL, American Medical Association, 2018. Available at: https://edhub.ama-assn.org/steps-forward/module/2702510 Accessed April 26, 2019.

Stair E: Stigma affects everyone, even doctors. National Alliance on Mental Illness (blog), October 18, 2017. Available at: https://www.nami.org/Blogs/NAMI-Blog/October-2017/Stigma-Affects-Everyone-Even-Doctors. Accessed April 5, 2019.

Stanford Medical Center: WellMD professional fulfillment model. Well MD, Stanford Medicine (website), 2019. Available at: https://wellmd.stanford.edu/center1.html. Accessed April 4, 2019.

Trockel M, Bohman B, Lesure E, et al: A brief instrument to assess both burnout and professional fulfillment in physicians: reliability and validity, including correlation with self-reported medical errors, in a sample of resident and practicing physicians. Acad Psychiatry 42(1):11–24, 2018 29196982

World Health Organization: Burn-out an "occupational phenomenon": International Classification of Diseases. Mental Health, World Health Organization, May 28, 2019. Available at: https://www.who.int/mental_health/evidence/burn-out/en. Accessed June 19, 2019.

Yellowlees P: Physician Suicide: Cases and Commentaries. Washington, DC, American Psychiatric Association Publishing, 2018

Chapter 3

A UNIFIED MISSION

Scenario

The silver sport utility vehicle meandered down the gravel driveway, tossing dust and loose stones into the otherwise peaceful summer morning. Pulling out onto the narrow road ahead, the driver caught a glimpse of his whitewashed, sprawling house, surrounded by his cherished garden. He had spent the past 10 years planting, pruning, and caring for a true country garden full of roses, verbena, and lavender. The trees lining the edges were weighted with full crops of oranges and cherries. His real prize was the massive burgundy bougainvillea climbing across the entrance to the house. Dr. Jack Shaper took great pleasure in his lush garden, knowing his own sweat and hard work had gone into planting every plant and tree over many years. The perfume of his variegated roses lining the driveway permeated the air, making it harder for him to leave. What a contrast to the many childhood homes on military bases that he had lived in as an "army brat" moving around the world, changing homes and schools most years, learning that it was not worthwhile making friends because such relationships never lasted.

As he turned onto the road, he noticed his wife, Laura, in his rearview mirror, waving goodbye from the porch steps. As usual, Laura had been up for hours organizing their lives. A dedicated teacher at the local high school, she was able to leave for work half an hour after her husband of 20 years and had the convenience of taking their two relatively independent teenage children with her. He knew that she would go inside and have a second cup of coffee with them while they finished their inevitably hurried breakfast, valuable minutes that she enjoyed and that kept her abreast of their news and activities.

Like his wife, Dr. Shaper also valued and enjoyed this time of the morning. His drive to the large primary-care clinic where he had worked for the past decade usually took about 15–20 minutes. In previous years, he had generally put the car radio on for the journey, listening to the morning news or some favorite music. Since taking up the role of medical director a year before, he found he preferred silence and some quiet time to contemplate the daily issues he faced and the decisions he might have to make.

Dr. Shaper was a thoughtful and careful man in all that he did. Tall and slim, with graying hair and glasses, he was a physician straight out of central casting, always impeccably dressed in a range of conservative navy-blue suits. He drove with care, keeping just at the speed limit and giving himself plenty of space from other cars so that he would always have time to react and avoid collisions. During the course of his career he had seen too many patients injured, often permanently, in motor vehicle accidents and had had several fatalities from this cause among his patient panel as well, so he was determined not to become such a victim.

Driving through the country roads this morning, he was a little anxious as he ruminated about his 16-year-old daughter, Melanie, who was ready to start learning to drive. He and Laura had been trying to work out ways that they could put her off this activity for a year or so, because they were both very aware of the number of adolescent fatalities in car crashes. Tragically, two seniors at the high school had died in this way the year before, and he was contemplating telling Melanie about a motor vehicle accident in which he had nearly been killed when he was 19, when he had foolishly accepted a ride home from a drunken friend. He knew Laura planned to discuss the subject with Melanie on the way to school with her that day. As parents, they admitted they felt conflicted because Melanie was a responsible girl who wanted the freedom that driving would allow.

Within a few minutes, he reverted to his usual habit of going over the upcoming workday's meeting and patient schedule in his mind. Much of his focus at work was on improving the morale of the 40 staff members, including 10 physicians, who worked for him. He knew this was the single most important reason he had applied for, and been appointed as, the clinic medical director. His first meeting this morning was likely the most important interaction he would have that day, a mentoring session with Dr. Lindy Isla, one of the other primary care internal medicine physicians at the clinic. He liked Dr. Isla. Despite being a relative newcomer to the clinic, she had already shown herself to be a natural leader and an influential member of the overall clinic team. If he was going to be able to make the changes he wanted, he had to have her fully committed to them.

Dr. Shaper reflected on how different the atmosphere in the clinic was now, compared with a year ago, and thought about the changes that had already occurred. As much as anything, he felt they were the result of his deliberate strategy of encouraging staff turnover and a gradual generational change in attitudes throughout the clinic. Adding several younger and more flexible clinicians who understood and supported the emerging plans of his new leadership team had helped, and he counted Dr. Isla as one of his key recruits.

He rubbed his head and smiled ruefully to himself. To think that just over a year ago he had been one of the younger physicians in the clinic and had been so fed up with his work that he had applied to work elsewhere, even though he didn't really want to move from the area. Rather to his surprise, he had been offered a position as medical director in a large inner-city clinic two states away. At that time, he had been at the local clinic for more than a decade. The positive side of this tenure had been his ability to finally, for the first time in his life, live a stable existence in one home, with a loving family and the opportunity to put down roots in the local community, and in his garden! No more constant moves to another cheap condo as had happened in college and medical school. He liked the area, with its great climate, good schools, and cultural diversity, and he had found new friends through the golf club and his children's school. The downside to working at the clinic at a time during which staff turnover had been minimal, except for occasional retirements, was that he could sense the stagnation and lack of change. The medical director at the time, Dr. Tobin, although pleasant enough, had clearly just been waiting for her own retirement and was averse to innovations. She had made it clear to everyone that she opposed the modernization of medical practice and was not keen to resource or pay for the necessary equipment upgrades that other clinics of this size received as routine. She preferred what she called "old style" medicine, where the doctor was always the kingpin in the organization and patients' needs were not as often prioritized.

Dr. Shaper didn't regret any of the increasingly difficult confrontations that he and four other primary care colleagues had had with Dr.

Tobin that had led to his thoughts of leaving. She had nicknamed them the "changelings" and had belittled them openly in response to their attempts to suggest improvements to increase the morale of the staff. She had opposed these ideas by telling stories of her own training, recounting at length how she had always had to work 80-hour weeks at a minimum, with minimal support or backup from more senior physicians. She had seemed proud of telling everyone that medicine was not a job but a vocation, and that anyone who didn't agree should get out of the proverbial kitchen. Interestingly, Dr. Tobin couldn't see that she had become chronically burned out, even though this actually had been pointed out to her numerous times and had led to her spending as much time as possible on administrative issues to reduce her patient care hours. Dr. Shaper recalled the massive blowup that had occurred when she unilaterally decided to increase the size of every other doctor's panel of patients by 10% without giving them any extra support or time. By then, the disputes about clinical care and workloads had become so serious that he and his four colleagues threatened to resign *en masse*, all of them feeling very unsupported and fed up with having to finish their work at night and on weekends. This threat, and the fact that he already had another job offer, had led to frantic negotiations with the clinic owners and to the sudden "retirement" of Dr. Tobin, along with two of her main supporters and friends of many years—the clinic administrator and another senior physician.

And the rest is history, he thought to himself, recalling how he had been encouraged by several colleagues to apply for the vacant medical director position. His wife and daughters did not want to move, and it was they who had finally persuaded him to apply for the director position. What a year it had been. He had been surprised at how much the clinic owners, a large health chain, had supported him, even paying for him to attend a series of conferences and workshops to upgrade his knowledge and skills in management and leadership. He had insisted that he still work half-time seeing patients when he was in the clinic, and he was pleased that he had done this because it gave him the opportunity to really see what was going on at the ground floor. Several of his younger physician recruits had expressed their surprise at how much clinic work he did, but he was pleased that they said it gave him much more "street credibility," to use their term. He remembered how he and Laura had discussed this, and she had advised him to always remember that he was a doctor first, but that being a doctor didn't mean he had to—or could—do all of his administrative duties himself. She had encouraged him to recruit really good administrative support staff to ensure he would be able to get home at a reasonable time and stay fully connected with his family and outside interests.

As he rounded the corner, past the local government offices, and drove the last half-mile to the clinic, Dr. Shaper finished his morning reverie by smiling to himself at Laura's encouragement of his outside interests. He looked forward to asking her tonight if she had really expected his golf handicap to improve in parallel with taking up this new job at a clinic in crisis. He hadn't seen "golf handicap" as a marker of physician well-being in any of the academic literature he had read and wondered lightheartedly if it should be. He certainly acknowledged internally that part of the reason for his improved scores was that he was really trying hard to "walk the talk" of the whole clinic, where his staff were now strongly being encouraged and supported to have a fair work-life balance.

Dr. Shaper drove onto the clinic grounds and parked under the large sycamore tree where he knew his car would be partly protected from the constant heat of the day. He added an extra shade over the back window to protect his new golf bag and clubs, a recent birthday present from Laura, so that they would be in perfect condition for him to use in the nine-hole competition in which they were partnering at their community golf club that evening. He walked across the parking lot and entered the clinic, a stately two-story Spanish colonial in white stucco with wide arches, a covered external walkway on the ground floor, and slim windows to keep out the heat on the second floor, all finished off with red clay roof tiles. He felt proud of the refurbishment of the building, now nearly complete, and especially liked entering the main door to see the clinic's mission statement painted on the wall for patients and staff to see. The creation of this statement had been one of his early wins, and he thought the process of developing it had really brought staff and patients together. He stopped to read the words painted in tall letters in the main waiting room: "We provide high-quality health care and have trusting relationships with our patients to meet their needs."

As Dr. Shaper moved through the clinic, he made sure to speak to everyone he met, briefly acknowledging some, asking about their families or other personal interests; congratulating several; thanking others; and generally speaking or smiling in a positive, supportive way. He gradually made his way up to the administrative offices in a suite at the back of the second floor. No longer did the administrators have the largest rooms with a beautiful view at the front of the clinic; those rooms were now used for patient education, meetings, and groups. He arrived at the administrative suite, the only non–patient care area in the building, and entered his office, a well-appointed and professional room that could be used by other staff for private meetings when he was working in the clinic downstairs. He sat in one of the four soft, cushioned chairs and took out Lindy Isla's file. He wanted to review his notes on their past mentoring sessions prior to her arrival for this morning's meeting.

Five minutes later, Dr. Isla appeared in the open doorway. Her well-pressed white lab coat had her name embroidered on the pocket. A stethoscope hung around her neck.

"Come in, Lindy. It's good to see you. I hope all is well. Please sit down," said Dr. Shaper.

Dr. Isla entered, shut the door, and sat opposite Dr. Shaper. She looked calm and confident and smiled warmly at him.

"Good morning. I can't believe it's been a month since our last mentoring session, Jack. So much has been going on, and I know we've talked about a lot of the issues in the clinic meetings with other staff. Before we get into my career plans, which I know we planned to focus on today, can I quickly get your advice about a patient-care concern I have?"

Dr. Shaper was not surprised at his junior colleague asking for advice about a patient before focusing on herself and her own needs. Only 2 years out of her internal medicine residency and fellowship in endocrinology, she was without doubt the endocrine-medicine expert in the clinic. With his encouragement, she was already overseeing the management of all the clinic's patients who had diabetes and other related endocrine disorders. Much of this was being done via e-consultations in the electronic medical record (EMR), with the aim that all diabetic patients treated in the clinic would ultimately be reviewed by her. The difficulty came when she inevitably found poor medical practice among some of the other physicians and had to tactfully suggest alternative treatment regimens to them, and sometimes she needed his support in this. Not surprisingly, her need for advice today was not really for a technical clinical problem but about how she could best improve the medication regimen that one of the few remaining older, long-term physicians in the clinic was prescribing for a patient, without offending their colleague.

As they finished discussing her concern, Dr. Shaper reflected on how clinically effective she was being; the average hemoglobin A1c, the best measure of diabetic control, of all the patients with diabetes treated at the clinic had dropped by more than a point since Lindy had begun her routine reviews only 6 months earlier. He decided to ask more about this result, because he knew that she was fascinated by these sorts of group outcomes.

"I am interested in how you think your work with our diabetic patients is coming along, and if we are giving you enough time for this indirect patient work?" he asked. "It seems to me that by having you electronically oversee everyone with endocrine disorders—even though most patients stay with their usual doctors—that you're being much more effective as a physician because you're affecting so many more patients than if you were personally treating them all. Am I right in that impression?"

"I'm sure you're right, Dr. Shaper, and I think this is a great way to work. It's much more enjoyable, and it keeps me interested and connected with all the other providers in the clinic."

He was curious. "What do you mean by 'more enjoyable'?"

"Well, you know how you've given me 8 hours of administrative time per week to do all my e-consults? I have found three really interesting aspects to them. First, I feel I get to know the patients through the EMR doing these asynchronous consultations, because they do indirectly affect the patients. It's also really helped me learn to use the EMR better. Second, the cases are academically interesting, and because I don't have to collect all the information myself, I spend most of my time analyzing the problem, which is often the part of the consultation that gets lost when you are seeing a patient in person. You have more time to think about the whole patient when working like this. And third, and most surprisingly to me, the e-consults are more relaxing to do, and I look forward to doing them. I've divided up the 8 hours you allocated into four 2-hour blocks of time, and I do them after lunch 4 days per week. As you know, that postnoon hour is always the most difficult time in terms of concentration. Now I can sit in my office and focus on patient problems while at the same time playing some of my favorite music through my headset. You cannot imagine how much more fun it is to solve problems to the music of Bach or Adele. I really look forward to my e-consult sessions and actually find them relaxing and interesting. That *has* to be good for my personal health, which is something I keep hearing you stress to all of us."

"That is really interesting," replied Dr. Shaper. "I must say, I hadn't thought of using technology in this way as being good for your personal well-being. Everyone just assumes that using the EMR is an added stress, as it certainly was here in the clinic when documentation took up so much extra time. It's good to see another positive side to all the technology changes we've been making. I wonder if you could continue collecting data on our patients with diabetes and then eventually publish the results? Would you be interested in doing that? It's certainly something that would be helpful from your career perspective."

Dr. Shaper watched Dr. Isla for her reaction to this suggestion. He wasn't quite sure how she would respond, because she certainly wasn't always keen to take up his suggestions, especially if they might involve her doing extra work outside of her usual clinic time. Not for the first time, he thought about the massive difference in attitudes between many physicians of his generation and those of Dr. Isla's, and he tried to understand this and put it in perspective. He knew that their age difference was about 20 years, but he was still trying to figure out all the differences in their approaches to work and their lifestyles. He was aware that he had never been good at developing and maintaining relationships in the professional setting and had only retained regular contact with two of his old medical school colleagues. He admired Dr. Isla for her medical knowledge and care, for the respect that the non-physician providers had for her, and for her obvious leadership skills. She had already demonstrated the capacity to speak up and lead debates among her colleagues in the clinic and to potentially act as an agent of change. She made him reflect on his own attitudes and experiences and on how he would have jumped at any opportunity like this had it been offered to him early in his career. His training at medical school and in residency had been so different from hers, killing his curiosity and forcing him to obey his attending physicians, not question them. How well he recalled the traditional educational mantra of "see one, do one, teach one" that had dominated his early career and that he now knew had led to so many mistakes and variations in practice.

He felt somewhat awkward and somehow intimidated in the presence of this assertive young woman who was so different from him. He regretted that thus far he hadn't been able to get to know her at a personal level as much as he would like, and he thought she raised barriers to her personal life whenever nonwork topics were raised. He knew she was very close with her family, who lived on the East Coast. He had no idea if she had significant interests or hobbies beyond the clinic's occasional in-house social gathering, which she always attended. She certainly seemed to get on well with the other younger staff in the clinic, and he had the impression they sometimes socialized together. He did know, however, that she guarded her personal time closely and almost never came to any clinic meetings if they were outside of usual work hours, and she was clear that she did not want to do any medical work at home beyond her routine on-call activities. He found this side of her frustrating, because throughout his career he had always been prepared to do extra voluntary work to help out wherever he was working, and because he felt it was expected by his senior colleagues and part of being a doctor.

"Thanks for the suggestion, Jack," Dr. Isla replied. "I agree with you and think that would be an interesting project. We need to talk about it some more, because I've never taken the lead on a full scientific paper, although I was included as a coauthor on a couple of short papers when I was a resident. What sort of paper were you envisaging?"

"I thought it could perhaps be your major project for your mentee annual development plan, which I wanted to discuss today anyway," he answered. "We would obviously have to plan this carefully and make sure you were able to collect the data properly. I have a colleague at the university who could also assist with statistics if necessary."

"What about actually writing the paper?" she asked. "The one thing I've found about research is that it always takes a lot longer than anyone originally expects. It's the time involved I would need to be careful about."

"You're right, of course. It's almost impossible to quantify how much time is ever going to be involved in a project like this, but I'm happy to help you with the data analysis and writing to take some of the load off."

"That's very kind of you, and I know I have a lot to learn in this area that you can help me with. I wonder if it would be possible for me to have some extra time in the clinic to work on this paper?" She looked Dr. Shaper directly in the eye. "After all, if the paper describes the work of the clinic, it would be good publicity for the clinic itself."

Dr. Shaper sighed inwardly. Dr. Isla had gone down the path he had thought she might take, and he knew he was going to have to refuse this request. He felt he was already being very generous giving her 8 hours per week for the e-consultations, and he couldn't justify reducing her direct patient care time any more at present because it would be too costly to the clinic and might be seen as favoritism by the other medical staff.

"I understand why you're asking for that, but I can't justify extra time for this write up, at least initially. If you're able to demonstrate that what you're doing is definitely improving patient care and is making us as a clinic more clinically and cost effective, then it's certainly something we could revisit in the future." He paused. "There are lots of ways you can do this write up, which I can help you with, and we are only talking about one paper over the course of a year, so it's not likely to take too much time per week. I can show you a number of ways you can work on the writeup during your usual work week. Would this work?"

Dr. Isla chose her words carefully. "First of all, I want to make it clear that I greatly appreciate your offer to help work with me on this. My major concern is quite simple. I just want to make sure that I'm not taking on something that I will not be able to do really well without putting in a whole lot of time outside of work. As you know, I'm a bit of a perfectionist, and I try to make sure that I succeed in everything I do, so I want to be really sure that I'm not overcommitting myself."

"I completely understand what you're saying, Lindy." He thought her response was actually more positive than he had been expecting and decided to try a middle road to ensure she was able to both commit to the project and succeed in writing the paper. "I think we can work this out. Let's use this as your major career development project for the year, so we can do a lot of the planning and organizing during our regular mentorship sessions. I'm sure we can fit a few extra of these in at mutually convenient times if necessary. It will be easy enough for you to add the project to the first draft of your individual development plan we're about to review. I'll work with you on a process for collecting all the data, which I am sure you can do during your current 8-hour allocation. Then we can arrange for you to take a professional writing course at the university, which the clinic will pay for and which can be done in your professional development education time allocation. The beauty of that course is that they insist you write up a real paper during the course, so you can use this topic as your course paper if we get the timing right and have your data collected beforehand."

"That sounds like a good process," Dr. Isla replied. "It sounds a bit like the one you arranged with Dr. Roberts, who told me about your work with him on evaluating our palliative care program. He's really excited about it and is already doing a lot of extra reading for the literature review. I just want to make it clear that I feel strongly about keeping definite boundaries between my work and my social life, so I won't be doing as much after hours as he is. I guess my project may just take a little longer."

"I understand and respect your views, Lindy, and am very aware of the importance of work-life balance. I think that is important for all of us. Let's spend the rest of the session going over your individual development plan, because I would like to focus on the clinical and educational goals you have for the coming year and how you will fully achieve them without burning yourself out."

At the end of the session, after Dr. Isla had left, Dr. Shaper reflected on how he felt the mentoring session had gone. He was not completely comfortable with his own performance, although he believed he had managed to impart appropriate advice without being too heavy handed. He had always found Dr. Isla a somewhat difficult person to mentor and wasn't quite sure why. He knew part of it was her wish to be so private and to not tell him much about her home or personal life. He tried hard not to be intrusive, but the result was that he felt he was giving career advice to someone he did not fully understand and whom he felt did not trust him greatly. He just wasn't sure why this was, and he hoped he wasn't being biased against her in any way, although he knew this was possible at an unconscious level. Was it a cultural or a generational issue, or both? A married, middle-aged male trying to communicate with a young, single female raised a lot of potential barriers, even if they were in the same profession and workplace. He fully understood how both he and Dr. Isla had their own implicit biases, how different her life experiences had likely been from his, and how she consequently had differing attitudes and communication styles. He knew this all made him slightly more reserved and hesitant with her than he had been with other junior mentees and worried it might lead to him not giving her the best advice or direction. He decided he just had to keep the relationship going as best he could so as to succeed in his mentoring role and help Dr. Isla in her career development. He concluded that his slightly reserved and nonintrusive approach was probably best for now because it gave her more time to get to know him and, he hoped, to learn to trust him.

Dr. Shaper snapped himself out of his reverie and turned back to his desk, checking his schedule on his computer. He had an hour to spare before the biweekly clinic staff meeting that he chaired, and he decided to go over the agenda carefully to make sure he was fully prepared. He was pleased that his three major original initiatives, the clinic strategic plan development, implementation of routine mentoring for all staff (including physicians), and the initial increased staff turnover, were no longer the main focus of the meeting. Instead, the first item on the agenda, titled *Huddle Implementation*, was a change he was determined to make to improve teamwork throughout the clinic and, consequently, the quality of patient care.

Dr. Shaper had learned a lot about huddles, a core component of Lean Six Sigma Accreditation. In the past year he had visited several primary-care clinics where they had been implemented. He had spoken to some of the authors of the American Medical Association's (2015) "Steps Forward" educational paper on implementing a daily team huddle and had become convinced that this was the fourth major innovation he needed to implement in the clinic and that, with the other changes already in process, now was the right time. He had discussed the beginning clinic-wide daily team huddles in his small management group over the past few months and had educated his colleagues about the importance of this approach. He was only too aware that the clinic had been operating in the past as though all the providers and staff were isolated individuals. As a result, they were often inefficient and slow, with key staff ignorant of daily patient or administrative changes and with little intraclinic communication. His main goals for this change were to improve communication by developing a more engaged workforce that he hoped would have a stronger team culture. The evidence from clinics that had introduced such huddles showed that they aligned the clinic team at the start of each session, allowed them to prospectively plan for patients who required extra time and assistance, and helped them prepare in advance for any staff, provider, or equipment changes during the day. A side effect of huddles that he hoped would occur in his clinic was improved morale of all staff; he knew that if the process occurred well, they would feel more in control of their work environment and be more knowledgeable about the clinic generally. Dr. Shaper reflected on the importance of today's meeting as the first official discussion about implementing huddles in the clinic. He knew the staff had heard about this from the management team, but they had not heard directly from him as to what he hoped to achieve from the huddles and how they would occur.

Dr. Shaper, well organized as usual, brought up his prepared PowerPoint presentation where he covered the evolution and rationale for huddles as well as their transition into health care from the auto industry, where they were first developed. His presentation then reviewed the practical implications of the daily 5- to 10-minute team meetings that now would occur at the beginning of every clinic day and the importance of the huddle process itself. He thought about what questions would be asked and tried to predict them. He could confidently expect that some staff would object to a daily meeting on the grounds that they were already short on time. Others would see this as just an administrative tool of little value and would complain about their perception of increased bureaucracy that might take time away from direct patient care. He and his management group had discussed these two issues and had developed good responses to these predictable objections to change. He just hoped that most of the staff would be prepared to give this innovation a try, even if it took several meetings to educate them. He would tell the group to expect an e-mail from him today with the American Medical Association's paper that described this whole process. He thought about his "plan B" if major objections arose—he would bring in clinicians and staff from other clinics that had implemented huddles and send some of his staff to other clinics to observe huddles in action.

He sat back and reviewed the agenda. He would focus entirely on huddles today so as to allow the staff as much discussion time as they wished. This would be yet another big change for them, and he had heard mutterings about "change toxicity" from some of his colleagues. He felt confident, however, that he would be successful in this specific initiative, and he remembered the words of the director of one of his recent leadership courses, who had advised him strongly to always focus on the early adopters of any change so that they could convince the bulk of the recipients that the change was helpful. He had never forgotten how this teacher had talked scathingly about "change laggards" whom he had described as the 10% of any group that will object to anything new you suggest and whom he thought should simply be ignored until they either gave up complaining or left. At the time, he had thought this view overly cynical, but his experience in the past year at the clinic had backed up what he had learned; several of the clinic's most resistant staff had voluntarily left or retired.

Dr. Shaper picked up his papers and his flash drive and, pausing only to put on his jacket and straighten his tie, left his office. He walked casually toward the clinic meeting room. Along the way he was joined by Dr. Isla and two of the other junior medical staff, all carrying the ubiquitous Starbucks coffee cups that seemed to be a permanent addition to their uniforms. He wondered to himself, not for the first time, how they managed to seemingly have permanently available coffee. He had never worked out where they found the time to buy the drinks. He rapidly put those thoughts aside as he reached the meeting room and moved to his place at the head of the conference table.

Most of the staff were already present, and a few stragglers followed Dr. Shaper in, so that within a few minutes he decided he should start the meeting. He looked around the room. A blur of matte white and beige walls, ceiling, and furnishings made it clear that this was a very utilitarian place, complemented by the six wooden tables placed together to form a single conference tabletop in the center of the room. Most of the staff present were female, with only four or five males spread around the room, and all wore scrubs of gray, blue, or white to identify their clinical roles. Dr. Shaper looked at Doug, his administrative assistant, and Polly, the clinic manager, who both sat to his right, and saw that they were ready to assist with note taking and questions. He looked up and addressed the group.

"It's great to see you all today. Thanks for coming to the clinic meeting. I was looking in my calendar earlier today and realized that this is an important day for me. I wonder if you can guess why that is?"

"Is it your birthday?" asked one of the nurses.

"No."

"Is it your wedding anniversary?" asked another.

"No. But you're getting closer. It is some sort of anniversary. Think about the clinic and what we are doing here."

The room went quiet as everyone thought about the question. Doug suddenly smiled and looked triumphant, turning toward Dr. Shaper. "I think I know. You were made medical director here a year ago. Is that it?"

"Well done, Doug. I had a funny feeling you would be the one who would work out the answer. After all, you have been here with me the same amount of time and have helped implement so many of the changes." Dr. Shaper smiled. "So, what I thought I would do, apart from inviting you all to a celebration of our clinic at 5 o'clock tonight in this room, is to briefly summarize some of the successes that we have achieved together over the past year. Then we will get on with the main topic of this meeting, which is the introduction of daily huddles throughout the clinic that I plan to commence next month. I hope that will be interesting to all of you and will help everyone realize that we are part way through a journey that's going really well and is designed to meet the mission of the clinic that I see every time I walk in our front door. I'm very proud of all of you for developing our mission statement, and the rest of our strategic plan, and I invite you to look at the back of the room behind me where it is painted on the wall."

Dr. Shaper turned and read off the wall: "We provide high quality health care and have trusting relationships with our patients to meet their needs."

He turned back to the group. "I have always liked that mission statement because it emphasizes both the high-quality care we provide and the relationships we build with patients. You all know that I feel very strongly that good, trusting relationships are a two-way street and that they are impossible if clinicians are not feeling healthy, comfortable, and motivated in their work. Many of you have heard me use the term 'joy' as something we are putting back into our work. If we've had one big success as a clinic over the past year, it is that I believe we've gone a long way toward putting joy back into our daily work lives, our patient relationships, and our relationships with each other. I personally feel that every time I come here. I feel positive and excited to be working with all of you and honored to be your leader. I know we all have bad days and personal difficulties, but for me, the biggest accomplishment for us to celebrate is our increased joy as we do really important and meaningful work as well as we can. I have no doubt in my own mind that we will continue to improve as a group, but I especially want to thank you all for the work you do and for your ability to listen and to run with some of the changes we have implemented, even though not all of them have succeeded."

Dr. Shaper looked around the group, who were listening intently. No one was eating or drinking. All had their eyes on him. "Before I go on, I wonder if someone might like to comment on this issue of joy, and in particular, how you feel yourselves about working here?"

Dr. Isla, who was sitting with a small group of the younger physicians at the far end of the table, put her hand up. "Thanks for asking, Dr. Shaper. Before I say anything else, I do want to congratulate you on your first year and make it clear that this is a great place to work, and I think that it will only continue to get better. I love the way you promote gratitude as a concept, so this is me showing gratitude to you. Thank you."

Dr. Shaper looked at Dr. Isla, somewhat worried about what might come next. He knew she was never afraid to speak up in public and had a habit of sometimes making comments that were not always well considered and would have been better raised during mentoring sessions.

She went on. "But I do want to emphasize one issue, and I hope we can talk about this more over the course of future meetings. You are always very strong about supporting all of us in having a good work-life balance and in keeping ourselves healthy and resilient. That's great. I really love the yoga class offered at the clinic twice a week and the mentoring processes we all have now. But although all that is good, it's still my impression that we're being asked to do more and more and to work more efficiently. That's going well at present, but what will happen if some of us run out of steam with all the changes going on? When we take on new things, we need to stop something else to make time."

Dr. Shaper breathed an inward sigh of relief. He was actually pleased that Dr. Isla had brought up this issue in the group, because it was also a real concern of his and something that he had thought about a lot, especially after their discussion this morning. "Thanks indeed, Lindy. As usual, you are able to correctly identify potential threats to what we're doing, and I thank you for that. I also really like that you are prepared to be so constructive in public, because I bet you have at least a partial answer to your own question ready. Am I right?"

Dr. Isla laughed. "You know, one of the really good things about working here, Dr. Shaper, is the way you ask us for our opinions—the way you listen to us even when we may be critical or not understand exactly what you want from us. I do want to suggest several improvements that I believe will make life easier for some of us providers, while at the same time improving patient care. But we've already discussed some of these privately, and I don't want to derail this meeting; I know you have a lot to discuss."

"That's okay, Lindy, why don't you share one of the ideas that you would like us to consider and that you think might make life easier for individual providers?"

She smiled. "I think as a clinic we should be exploring using virtual care technologies much more than we do at present. That will allow us to see patients either in person or online and to develop a hybrid relationship with them, as is happening at a number of other health systems. We could even potentially sometimes work from home rather than come into the clinic. This approach would really help the many parents who work here, and it might actually allow us to have longer clinic hours and to be open electronically at nights and on weekends when patients may at times prefer to be seen." Dr. Isla stopped talking and looked inquisitively at Dr. Shaper.

Dr. Shaper nodded. "I agree with you completely, and I have that issue on my list of potential innovations for the next year. I would personally like to be able to see some of my own patients from home, maybe one evening per week, because then I could get some more golf in on a free afternoon! I have some patients who find it difficult to take time off from their jobs during the day. Let's talk more about that suggestion. That may even be an area you would like to work on, along with your work on e-consults, which of course could also be done at home."

Dr. Shaper, relieved at the positive outcome from this interaction, turned to the group again and got back to his original agenda.

"Before we start discussing huddles and improving our communication throughout the clinic, I just want to briefly reiterate what I see as our major successes this year and to thank you all for your work on them. First is our unified mission. I mentioned our mission statement, but it is so impressive that you all really seem to live this mission and are proud of it. We had a lot of discussion to arrive at this, but that was very helpful, and although a few people disagreed and thought I was being overly bureaucratic, I do hope that most of you feel really invested in what we do."

Dr. Shaper looked around the room and stopped to emphasize this point. He noted a lot of positive looks and nods of heads and continued. "Second, I really do believe we are changing the culture of the clinic and that you are all much more involved in decision making and in what we do. I have always found it much more rewarding to work in an environment where I not only know what is going on but also have some influence over what happens, so I think posting all our meeting notes online has been excellent. And if someone misses a meeting, they can keep up to date easily. It's good to see how many of you attend relevant meetings and give constructive feedback whenever necessary. I get to hear the great majority of your ideas, and we try hard to implement as many as necessary. Incidentally, before I forget, a few of you asked if we could put in electric vehicle charging stations, and you will be glad to hear that four of these are going in very soon for use by anyone who works or attends here." A rustle of appreciation passed through the room, and a couple of staff members spontaneously applauded. "Thank you. I am waiting in line for a new Tesla myself, and I hope we will increase the number of these spaces in the future, while including this in our energy-saving strategies that many of you have been advocating.

"Our next major initiative has been the development of more efficient workflow throughout the clinic, including the rooming process and scheduling, as well as giving our patients access to parts of their EMRs and the ability to securely message providers. This has allowed all of us to work to the top of our professional licenses much more than previously, which makes life much more interesting and rewarding. I thank all of you for constantly improving these processes, because improving our workflow is going to be a never-ending job and may also be changed yet again when we introduce more virtual care, as Lindy just suggested.

"Finally, last but certainly not least, is the push we have had to provide mentoring for more and more staff. I know we're only part way through this initiative, but I'm already hearing really good things from those of you who've been developing your own individual development career plans. I hope that our mentoring program will eventually become one of the core infrastructure programs on which the clinic is built. I do hope you all take your mentoring relationships, as mentor or mentee, seriously, and get as much out of them as you can." Dr. Shaper looked at his watch and decided to move on. "Time is getting on, and I want to have a really good discussion about our internal and clinical communications and the use of daily huddles. Polly, as clinic manager, you've been mainly driving this issue, with your background in Six Sigma training and certification, so perhaps you could lead this discussion."

Commentary

The clinic described in this scenario had been fairly run down and behind the times for several years. Not surprisingly, morale was low; staffing was difficult to maintain, as demonstrated in Dr. Shaper's case when he almost left; and clinical services most likely were mediocre. In this setting, any physicians who wanted to make changes were likely to leave, and levels of provider burnout across all health care disciplines, although not formally measured, would certainly have been at similarly high levels as measured in a number of institutions. My previous book (Yellowlees 2018) summarized the literature on burnout and its causes, and Shanafelt et al. (2015) identified that between 40% and 50% of doctors in large community surveys have at least one symptom complex of the three burnout-syndrome sets described in Chapter 2.

In this setting, Dr. Shaper had stepped in as the new medical director, determined to make a number of organizational changes that would improve the quality of care provided at the clinic while at the same time also improving the well-being of the providers and clinic staff to boost their morale and help them rediscover joy in medicine. The scenario hints that Dr. Shaper had a difficult childhood and medical training, and that his response has been to have a strong focus on stability and on working to improve both his home and work environments. Shanafelt and Noseworthy (2017) described a connection between physician burnout levels and quality of care, patient safety, physician turnover, and patient satisfaction. It is likely that Dr. Shaper reviewed the nine organizational strategies that those authors described and learned how to implement the goals of the three domains of the Stanford Wellness Framework (Stanford Medical Center 2019), both of which are discussed in Chapter 2. He then introduced several very specific changes in his first year running the clinic, seemingly with some considerable success. These comprised

1. Development of a shared mission
2. Improved communication and involving physicians and other providers in management decisions, thus improving their local knowledge and feeling of being influential and in control
3. Development of improved workflows and efficient practices
4. Placing a strong focus on mentoring and individual physician career development plans
5. Establishing individual and personal resilience supporting activities

This leads to two questions. First, what are effective ways of introducing change within a clinical environment, and second, why should these specific changes be likely to reduce burnout and improve patient care and safety?

Dr. Shaper's leadership director, as described in the scenario, had been talking about Rogers' (2003) seminal work on change management and the diffusion of innovations when he mentioned "early adopters" and "laggards." Although the first edition of Rogers' book was written almost 40 years ago, it is still highly relevant to anyone wanting to drive changes in an environment as complicated and regulated as health care, and his messages and techniques have been particularly successful in situations that require technology innovations. The core message from the change management literature is to carefully plan any initiatives or change projects, to involve a group of individuals who are committed and interested early on (the early adopters), and to run pilot projects with them to prove the effectiveness of the innovation internally. Once this is proved, have the early adopters—who will ideally be representative of as wide a range of professionals as possible—tell their colleagues and the rest of the workforce about their projects, in the knowledge that most of their colleagues will be prepared to change if appropriately persuaded. These internal "salespeople" will be much more effective than most outside experts, although some experts still may need to be brought in to validate the activity.

The critical issue about any change management initiative is to be aware that, inevitably, a small group of people will fight against it and try to undermine what is happening. It is crucial to be aware of this and to not let these individuals succeed. Sometimes it may be necessary to specifically identify them and work with them separately—or isolate them—so that they do not get too much of a stage to oppose ideas. That may sometimes even mean moving them to alternative areas or putting pressure on them to cease being disruptive. In the scenario, several individuals who would have been in that "laggard" group, as Rogers defined them, decided to leave the clinic, and in this situation where a lot of change was planned, that was probably the best result for both the individuals and for Dr. Shaper. Similar results have been seen with the introduction of the EMR over the past decade; a number of physicians have used their objection to learning such a new and sometimes awkward and time-consuming technology as a rationale to retire, rather than go through a difficult learning and change-related process.

The final step in any change process is to constantly communicate the outcomes; celebrate successes and reward those involved as positively as possible, as Dr. Shaper was doing with his after-clinic celebration; and evaluate the overall results. Then the cycle must begin again to determine if more changes can be made so that, ultimately, a change-friendly culture is developed.

Dr. Shaper used a lot of leadership approaches learned from industry, notably those promoted by Bob Chapman (Chapman and Sisodia 2015), a charismatic CEO who developed a number of leadership programs, which Dr. Shaper might have attended, that focused on his personal lifelong leadership learning. Chapman describes *leadership* as being the stewardship of the lives entrusted to you and notes that people want to know who they are and that they matter, as shown in the clinic meeting. This is in contrast to *management*, which he describes as a manipulative process. Instead Chapman promotes listening with empathy as a crucial skill and the most powerful act of caring and says that giving recognition and celebrating successes at work is essential. His other key theme, which Dr. Shaper adopts, is the similarity between parenting and leadership, with his view that all leaders should be the leader you want your children to have. So with this approach to leadership in mind, why should the five interventions that Dr. Shaper introduced in his first year reduce burnout, improve the well-being of the clinic workforce, and thereby improve the quality of care and patient safety parameters in the clinic?

First was the development of a shared mission. Why is this important? A mission statement provides a way of judging the overall success of an organization and its various programs and helps to verify that an organization is making the right decisions and is on the correct track. It is really a direction indicator within a strategic planning framework, and in most cases would certainly not be developed in isolation but as part of a wider strategic plan that would also include a vision, objectives, strategies, and action plans. Numerous websites cover strategic planning, and many consultants or educational experts are available who can assist in their development if required. In the scenario, this was Dr. Shaper's first initiative, and developing a strategic plan had allowed him to demonstrate his caring for his staff by getting groups of diverse clinicians and administrative staff together to start planning a new, alternative path for the clinic. This activity also gives physicians and all involved the opportunity to have real input into the direction and priorities of the clinic, something that is well known to be very important in improving morale and reducing burnout levels.

Thus, the mission statement and associated plans, and the process of development, have the very beneficial extra consequence of bringing staff together and giving them a greater sense of meaning and control over their workplace environment. We have all worked on projects on which everyone seems to be pulling in opposite directions, and the project ultimately fails. It seems a very basic requirement that everyone should understand why an organization exists, what products or services they produce, who their primary customers are, and what outcomes they hope to achieve. Dr. Shaper's focus on this as his first change initiative made a lot of sense, as did his promotion of the mission statement by having it painted in prominent places and regularly mentioning it in clinic presentations.

The second initiative was involving physicians and other staff more in management decisions, whether in specific committees or by just asking and listening to them and then taking action, such as with the electric vehicle charging stations. Shanafelt et al. (2017) wrote about the importance of the business case in investing in physician well-being, yet one of the most stressful situations for us all is feeling out of control, for whatever reason. Therefore, being included in decision-making processes and being constantly educated and brought up to date on what is happening throughout the work environment is not only settling for all but actually makes economic sense. Making sure that physicians and other staff are involved in committees and any decision-making processes as much as possible is not only good for the clinic but also for the health of the staff. A substantial literature is available on how feeling more in control at work, especially of personal time, improves productivity, reduces unwanted emotions, and leads to an improved professional reputation. One of the interesting concepts about the health care industry is that, unlike most Americans, two-thirds of whom report routinely in surveys that they dislike their jobs, the great majority of health care professionals, especially physicians, report that they enjoy their work and, in particular, find it meaningful. This is a very positive and important issue because it is extremely difficult to engage successfully with individuals who do not enjoy their work and who see little sense in it.

Dr. Shaper's third priority was developing improved clinical and business workflows and more efficient practices. There are many approaches to this. He mentioned improved use of EMRs, which are often cited as an extra stressor for clinicians (National Academy of Medicine 2019) but which, if used well with appropriate training in place, can dramatically improve patient care, particularly when delivered by teams. In the clinic, Dr. Shaper was focusing on having individual providers work at the top of their licenses. That likely would have involved having medical assistants or physician assistants room patients and perform initial documentation, allowing physicians and other high-level practitioners to take supervisory or analytic roles. These physicians then were likely to be less focused on taking basic information (e.g., required surveys and questionnaires) or reviewing medication lists and vital physical assessments and better able to concentrate on more difficult aspects of each patient's case. Moawad (2017) recently wrote about practicing at the top of a license, which she defined as "the idea that physicians often have to gain multiple certifications and that the top of the license is the certification that takes the longest to attain, has the highest number of prerequisites, allows a physician to perform procedures commanding the highest reimbursement or for which few are qualified." She identified five rationales for this approach:

1. Practice and experience: Patients benefit because doctors are constantly using and improving their knowledge and skills.
2. Working as consultants: Experts can assist other practitioners with difficult referrals.
3. Improved reimbursement: Higher certification should translate to being better paid for specialist skills and procedures.
4. Easier identification of roles: Tasks and procedures and who can perform them is more clearly delineated, which improves efficiency, instead of higher-level providers being expected to pick up the slack and fill gaps at disproportionate cost.
5. Payers gain: When as many people as possible are doing work that no one else on a lower pay scale can do, the overall cost of this work goes down, so clinics like Dr. Shaper's become more financially efficient.

The fourth area of innovation Dr. Shaper mentioned was to increase the emphasis on mentoring and mentee outcomes. This chapter features Dr. Shaper's perspective on mentoring and his uncertainties around his relationship with his younger mentee, Dr. Isla, who at times seemed to intimidate him, to a certain extent, with her confidence and differing generational expectations. The literature on mentoring is extensive across many professional and work-related areas, and the usual process is very much a two-way street, with benefits for both mentee and mentor. Dr. Shaper was clearly gaining some of the advantages for mentors that are widely described in the literature (Lyman 2016), including the ability to better understand and to learn from his mentees. In this instance, Dr. Shaper learned more about the capacity of technology to improve clinical care while being reminded that the lessons he had taught to Dr. Isla still also applied to him. At the same time, Dr. Shaper was able to gain a wider social perspective through his discussions with Dr. Isla and through examining and helping her with her projects, increasingly trying to see issues and problems through her eyes and not just his own. This, he hoped, then would enable him to improve his own leadership capacity, not just individually but also by working through Dr. Isla and having her influence changes in others. Mentoring is a key intervention and well-being process that appears in several case studies in this book, and Chapter 4 in particular has a stronger focus on mentoring, from Dr. Isla's perspective, with a more extended discussion in the commentary.

The fifth and final initiative Dr. Shaper had commenced at the clinic involved some specific resilience-enhancing activities for the staff. Although it is well known that it is impossible to "resilience yourself" out of burnout (Yellowlees 2018), resilience can be both learned and enhanced if the time and opportunity are available, and good evidence has shown that a range of individual and systemic changes are associated with reduced physician burnout over time (West et al. 2016). In the scenario, the resilience activity mentioned is the introduction of yoga classes at lunchtimes, but numerous other activities could have been considered. Dr. Shaper could have chosen from literally hundreds of different activities had he wanted to; I found more than 20 million hits on Google in response to the search phrase "resilience-enhancing activities." Had Dr. Shaper consulted the excellent Road to Resilience website set up by the American Psychological Association (2018), he would have found an impressive number of strategies and suggestions for increasing personal resilience, from mindfulness meditation to improved physical fitness and communication training. Similarly, he might have considered buying Southwick and Charney's 2018 book on resilience for his mentees, which focuses on evidence-based ways to boost individual emotional resilience. The book includes the following list of approaches:

1. Be optimistic.
2. Face your fears.
3. Have a moral compass.
4. Practice spirituality.
5. Get social support.
6. Have resilient role models.
7. Maintain physical fitness.
8. Be a lifelong learner.
9. Use a variety of coping strategies.
10. Find meaning in what you do.

All of these approaches are very helpful for individuals who wish to improve their own resilience. Given the task awaiting him in his new role, and with the amount of change he needed to create in the clinic, Dr. Shaper also might well have bought the book *Grit* (Duckworth 2018) for himself. In this book, Duckworth describes how the secret of achievement for anyone striving to succeed at a difficult task is not talent but what the author describes as "grit," a special blend of passion and perseverance. As medical director, a major part Dr. Shaper must play is acting as a role model for all other staff, and following the approaches described by Duckworth would help him not only succeed with his change goals but also be seen as an excellent active role model for medical leadership by his colleagues.

References

American Medical Association: Implementing a Daily Team Huddle. AMA Steps Forward (website). Chicago, IL, American Medical Association, 2015. Available at: https://edhub.ama-assn.org/steps-forward/module/2702506. Accessed June 26, 2018.

American Psychological Association: The Road to Resilience (website). Washington, DC, American Psychological Association, 2018. Available at: http://www.apa.org/helpcenter/road-resilience.aspx. Accessed July 18, 2018.

Chapman B, Sisodia R: Everybody Matters. New York, Penguin, 2015

Duckworth A: Grit: The Power of Passion and Perseverance. New York, Simon and Schuster, 2018

Lyman A: Why mentoring others has helped me. Huffington Post, May 31, 2016. Available at: https://www.huffingtonpost.com/alex-lyman/why-mentoring-others-has-_b_10214756.html. Accessed July 7, 2018.

Moawad H: Practicing at the top of your license. MD Mag, May 3, 2017. Available at: https://www.mdmag.com/physicians-money-digest/contributor/heidi-moawad-md/2017/05/practicing-at-the-top-of-your-license. Accessed July 16, 2018.

National Academy of Medicine: Action Collaborative on Clinician Well-Being and Resilience Knowledge Hub (website). Washington, DC, National Academy of Medicine, 2019. Available at: https://nam.edu/initiatives/clinician-resilience-and-well-being. Accessed April 3, 2019.

Rogers E: Diffusion of Innovations, 5th Edition. New York, Simon and Schuster, 2003

Shanafelt TD, Noseworthy JH: Executive leadership and physician well-being: nine organizational strategies to promote engagement and reduce burnout. Mayo Clin Proc 92(1):129–146, 2017 27871627

Shanafelt TD, Hasan O, Dyrbye LN, et al: Changes in burnout and satisfaction with work-life balance in physicians and the general US working population between 2011 and 2014. Mayo Clin Proc 90(12):1600–1613, 2015 26653297

Shanafelt TD, Goh J, Sinsky C: The business case for investing in physician well-being. JAMA Intern Med 177(12):1826–1832, 2017 28973070

Southwick S, Charney D: Resilience: The Science of Mastering Life's Greatest Challenges. Cambridge, UK, Cambridge University Press, 2018

Stanford Medical Center: WellMD professional fulfillment model. Well MD, Stanford Medicine (website), 2019. Available at: https://wellmd.stanford.edu/center1.html. Accessed April 4, 2019.

West CP, Dyrbye LN, Erwin PJ, et al: Interventions to prevent and reduce physician burnout: a systematic review and meta-analysis. Lancet 388(10057):2272–2281, 2016 27692469

Yellowlees P: Physician Suicide: Cases and Commentaries. Washington, DC, American Psychiatric Association Publishing, 2018

Chapter 4

TRUST, MENTORING, AND INNOVATION

Scenario

Lindy Isla sat on a barstool, leaning over the granite countertop in the kitchen of her condo. She was already dressed in her favorite blue running gear and shoes. She felt energized just looking forward to her morning run down by the river. Suddenly, the ringing of her cellphone interrupted her plan. She clicked as soon as she saw it was her mom calling via video chat.

"Hey, Mom! It's good to hear from you. How are you and Dad?"

"We're good, Honey," her mom replied. "And you look great."

"This is so much better, being able to actually see you as well as talk with you! You look great!" Dr. Isla spoke rapidly and enthusiastically, happy to speak to her parents even though it interrupted her prework routine. "I love your new haircut; I see why you decided to change to a new stylist. That's a really nice look for you. I see Dad has joined us, too! It's good to see you both."

"It looks like we interrupted you this morning, so I'm sorry about that." Mrs. Isla grew serious. "Your father and I thought we should make sure you know what's been happening with your Nana."

Lindy sat back, looking and feeling concerned. It was unusual for her parents to phone so early in the morning, even with the 3-hour time difference between the East and West Coasts. They usually tried hard not to interrupt her on workdays. She knew they were very proud of all she had achieved, being the first child in the large African American family to attend college and to get all the way through medical school as well. They were a loving family, and Lindy had always had a very close relationship with her parents, her two younger brothers, and her maternal grandmother, Nana, who had lived with her parents since Grandpa died 3 years earlier. The phone was the family lifeline, and they always spoke on weekends when everyone could relax and take their time. This call was odd, and Lindy had a feeling of foreboding about what was coming next.

"What's happening with Nana?" she asked. "Tell me everything."

"Well, we've all been worrying about Nana for a while. You know yourself how she's been getting more forgetful over the past year. I remember you asking us to take her to the doctor and get her fully checked out when you were here at Christmas. Nana is stubborn and always refused to go, but yesterday she suddenly became very confused and didn't know where she was for a few minutes. We finally ended up taking her to see Dr. Garcia, her primary care doctor, even though she was hesitant at first. Dr. Garcia has a good rapport with Nana, and he was very thorough. He did a physical and asked her a lot of memory questions, some of which she got wrong. He also ordered some lab tests on her. Anyway, after he had seen her, he invited us to join them. He spoke openly with all three of us and told us that he thinks she probably has early dementia. Nana admitted she knew she was getting more forgetful over the past year and was not really surprised. I know you've been concerned about her forgetfulness for a while."

Lindy saw the strain and the worried looks on her parents' faces. Her mom was almost in tears, and Lindy knew they needed her to be strong and helpful, however upset she felt. This was the role she had played in the family for as long as she could remember; everyone called her the "family's doctor." Her large extended family, mostly spread across the East Coast, certainly treated her that way, always contacting her about problems, medical or otherwise, for her advice and help. She understood that they did this out of respect for her achievements, and that at one level the frequent requests for help were a compliment to her, but she did find them wearing on occasions.

Not this time. Lindy had always been very close to her Nana. It was Nana who had instilled in her the sense of confidence to work hard and to succeed beyond her wildest dreams at college, and Nana who had pushed her to go on to medical school. It was Nana who had read to her from an early age and had instilled a love of books and lifelong learning. Nana had been there through the ups and downs of her teen years, always guiding her to focus on her dream of becoming a doctor. She had taught Lindy the importance of hard work, self-respect, and making the most of her many talents. Although Lindy loved everyone in her family, Nana was her rock.

She held the phone up before her so her parents could see her better. "I'm so sorry to hear that, Mom. Give Nana my love. How is she today? How are you and Dad dealing with this news? Is Nana there at the moment? Can I speak to her?" Her rush of questions spilled out, showing her concern.

"She's still in bed this morning, sweetheart. I looked in on her before calling you because I knew you'd immediately want to speak to her, but she was asleep, so I didn't disturb her. She was really back to normal last night and seemed fine at dinner. I'm sure she would love to speak to you tonight if you can call after work." Her mother paused. "It's just more of a confirmation for us. I think we've both been expecting this but have avoided thinking about Mom's deteriorating memory, even though you made your concerns clear to us. We just cannot avoid this issue anymore and are going to have to think and plan how we may look after her in the future. For many years yet, I hope."

Lindy nodded. "That's right, Mom. I'm afraid there likely will have to be some changes in her care over time if she does have early dementia, but she should continue to be okay for the present. Most people deteriorate very slowly. Unfortunately, you can never predict how people are going to progress, how long they will remain independent, or even how independent they will be. Everyone is different. But Nana has always been a real fighter, so she'll likely take this as yet another challenge, once it's all explained to her." She became wistful. "I'm just sorry I'm so far away from you, and from her. After 9 months, I'm just starting to feel settled over here. I love my condo in particular, and even work is going better than it was originally. But this would be so much easier if I hadn't moved. I was about to send you and Dad some money to buy tickets so you could come out here to visit me again, but maybe we should put that on hold. I'll see if I can get a couple of days off to come back and see you all soon. I'd still love for you both to see where I live, and I hope someday you can visit and stay with me in my spare room. There's so much I would like to explore with you here. That may have to wait for now. I guess a lot will depend on Nana."

"Don't worry about that, please, Lindy," her father answered. "I think you made a good decision to move and to make your own life as a doctor. We're all so proud of you. Come back when you can, although I do hope we can make the trip out your way eventually. I think Nana will be fine left here if we can make arrangements for her while we're away; your brothers can stay with her. Anyway, we just wanted to make sure you're kept up to date. Go now and get on to work, and let's talk tonight, or this weekend if that's better for you. We will give Nana your love. And we love you. Bye for now."

"Goodbye Mom, goodbye Dad. I love you both," Lindy said, ending the conversation. She decided to still go out for a run, although now she only had time for a 3-mile circuit rather than the original 5-mile jog she had planned. Lindy looked around the condo. It had a very clean, simple look that she loved, with modern minimalist furniture, several pieces in white lacquer. The poster from the New Orleans Jazz Festival she had attended hung proudly over her mantle. Those 4 days in a New Orleans hotel, her flights, and her meals had all been paid for by Nana as a gift to Lindy for getting into medical school. A large window overlooked the river and the track she would be running on momentarily. She put her phone, keys, water bottle, and pepper spray canister into her small waist pack and checked to make sure her condo was tidy before leaving.

Lindy enjoyed running because it gave her time to think and plan. She was a thoughtful, organized person, rather compulsive at times, and very aware of protecting herself and making sure no one took advantage of her. She knew that her inherent defensiveness was perhaps excessive at times and gave her a reputation of being hard to get to know, as though she had a wall around herself. But as a black professional female who had seen and been the victim of all sorts of biases and discrimination in her life, she tended to take her time with trusting new people until she felt comfortable with them.

This morning she had two major issues to think about. First of all was Nana, and what her likely dementia would mean for her. She missed Nana greatly at the best of times, and moving across the country from her family had been very difficult, but overall it had been good for her confidence and independence. Now she wondered whether she should go back to the East Coast, not necessarily to Boston, but somewhere closer so that she could see more of Nana and help her in the future. She knew this would be a very difficult decision that she would have to make in the next year or so. In the meantime, she looked forward to speaking with Nana that evening and knew that she would be peppered with questions from her about her health and what might happen in the future. Nana was nothing if not direct and inquisitive, and she had been telling Lindy for years to be more open and trusting with her friends and colleagues, especially now that she was a full-fledged physician.

Although her Nana was of great concern to her, she found that she spent most of her run along the river on this sunny day planning for her monthly mentoring session with Dr. Shaper. This meeting was her immediate priority.

Lindy liked Dr. Shaper and thought she had a good working relationship with him. Certainly, he had been very helpful to her and had particularly supported her early attempts to work in a different way at the clinic and to use technology to do more consulting with other doctors about their endocrine patients. She acknowledged to herself what an improvement he had made in the clinic and how her life had become more professionally rewarding since she had started there. Still, she found it very difficult to have a good relationship with him as his mentee. She had actually gone as far as talking to Nana about this last Christmas and had been advised to open up a bit more herself. She knew she hadn't done this.

She thought about issues important to her that she felt unable to talk about with him. The first was simply the fact that she had found working at the clinic much harder than she had expected. She'd come to the clinic hoping to make an immediate impact, fresh out of her fellowship, and felt frustrated that she didn't really seem to have succeeded in this as much as she had hoped, although she knew it was early days yet, and that she was still going through the transition from resident to attending. She didn't feel she could tell Dr. Shaper this, however, because she saw it as a sign of her own weakness. He was working so hard to improve the clinic and clearly saw her as someone who could help him, but she wanted to move forward much more quickly than he seemed to appreciate, especially in changing how she practiced. She had recently begun to think that she was only at the clinic because of the debt relief program she was in that allowed her to work for 5 more years and pay off her entire student debt of $250,000. That debt hung over her like the sword of Damocles. She thought about it constantly and had had nightmares about it growing larger and smothering her. The system was so unfair, forcing people like her, who were from poor families with few resources, to develop such debt! This financial pressure, made worse by the need to constantly help members of her family, kept her working, but her frustration at being trapped in such a financial situation was the major reason she did what she considered only a fair amount of work, and little more, at the clinic.

She knew Dr. Shaper was equally frustrated with her for setting such strong work boundaries and refusing to do extra work outside of clinic hours, but she thought this was the only way she could maintain control of a situation in which she felt unfairly constrained by financial pressures. She was exploring doing an MBA[1] program online as well as researching other jobs after hours, and she was constantly being approached by recruiters. She dreamed of finding a job where she could reduce her clinical work and combine it with more preventive teaching and educational activities in the community, but none of those jobs matched the financial and debt relief package she had at the federal clinic.

Another issue acted as a block in her relationship with Dr. Shaper as well. She'd thought about this a great deal and had decided that it really came down to her lack of trust in him. She didn't blame him for this, but she had thought and read about mentor-mentee relationships and knew that they could be fraught with difficulty. This concern was why she had told him almost nothing about her personal life and why he, even after several mentoring sessions, still had no real idea about what she did outside the clinic. She certainly wouldn't tell him about Nana's situation, despite how upset she was this morning. He had been trying subtly to find out about her over the course of their meetings, asking questions about what she was doing on the weekend or what television shows she liked. He had talked about movies he had seen and places he had visited to find out if she had also been there. He had even talked about his wife and what they did together on one occasion.

She rebuffed all of his attempts. What she had thought a lot about was *why* she didn't trust him. She knew she had had similar reactions to other male mentors in the past and had always found females much easier to communicate with. She had no doubt it was partly a gender issue and that, as a woman, she found it easier to connect with other women who had had similar professional experiences. She had read a lot about implicit bias and how it impacted characteristics such as race and gender, which she knew applied to both Dr. Shaper and to herself, but she thought that this was also something she could not possibly discuss with him. What about the difference in their ages? He was much younger than her father, certainly, but at times he came across to her paternalistically, which she found offensive, although she knew it was not deliberate. So, she saw barriers to trust around age, gender, and race. These seemed like too much to overcome, never mind acknowledging them to

---

[1]MBA=Master of Business Administration.

Dr. Shaper. As a seemingly genuinely nice and caring man, he would probably be highly offended if she brought her concerns out in the open.

As she finished her run and walked the last 100 yards uphill to her condo, she couldn't see any way through these barriers except to continue on as she had been and remain a closed book to Dr. Shaper. With today's news about Nana, on top of her own ambivalence about work, she decided she was right to continue to perform adequately at the clinic but would not take on any additional work, especially unpaid work.

After showering and drinking a healthy smoothie that she had made for breakfast, Lindy rapidly scanned the overnight e-mails on her phone for anything urgent. She found mainly notes from political and medical organizations such as the American College of Endocrinology and the National Medical Association, the latter advertising their upcoming national conference, which she hoped to attend. She had two e-mails from recruiters, and neither looked interesting. She wished the recruiters would indicate where the positions were actually based instead of giving meaningless, overly positive descriptions of the environments. Putting her phone away, she left the condo and hopped into her 4-year-old Honda, aiming directly for the nearest Starbucks. The radio played her favorite jazz channel, which reminded her of the clubs in Boston she had frequented while at college. She arrived at the clinic 15 minutes later, carrying her carefully made grande latte, and went to her office.

As usual, Lindy was in before any patients were booked to arrive so that she could review her patient list for the day and respond to any urgent patient requests. She noticed that the inbox for her EMR[2] had about 60 messages in it, which was not as bad a start to the day as it could have been but still meant at least 1–2 hours' solid work that she had to fit in around her patient load. Her first patient was not scheduled until after her mentoring session with Dr. Shaper. She noted another gap in her schedule around lunch for the monthly clinic meeting. She wanted to review her independent development plan (IDP), which she brought up on the computer.

Lindy had been opposed to the whole concept of the IDPs when Dr. Shaper had introduced them. She had been fortunate to have two really helpful mentors previously, one while she was at medical school and another when she was a resident, and neither had been very formal or insisted on documenting her career plans and directions. She had always thought the most important part of mentoring was having someone lis-

---

[2]EMR=electronic medical record.

ten to her and occasionally gently advise her about possible alternative approaches to the one she was considering. Both of her other mentors had been women, however, and Dr. Seview, her residency training director, had also been black. She had felt much more comfortable with them and more prepared to discuss intimate and personal issues. She was still in regular contact with Dr. Seview by e-mail and phone, and she was the only person Lindy felt really understood her and with whom she had discussed her current feelings about her job and Dr. Shaper. She actually had been quite surprised when Dr. Seview backed up Dr. Shaper's comments about the importance of IDPs, and because of Dr. Seview's encouragement, she had finally put a draft IDP together.

Lindy started to review her IDP on the screen in front of her, immediately wondering how different it might be were she to find a new job somewhere else. Perhaps she would simply have to make that sort of move anyway if Nana deteriorated significantly. In the meantime, she read through her draft IDP, which Dr Shaper wanted to discuss today.

Identify Personal and Institutional Long-Term Goals

Why did you decide to work at the clinic?

I like the mission of the clinic, looking after a diverse and frequently underserved community, and I want to be able to educate them and eventually become part of their community, perhaps in some leadership role using my medical skills. I am academically very interested in diabetes, and because the clinic population is heavily afflicted by this illness, I would like to do some research to find out more about how to help them, perhaps using a range of virtual-care approaches.

What do you personally hope to accomplish in your career?

Specific Goals in Focus Areas

1. Clinical Care

Year in review: I believe I am providing good-quality individual care and have started to electronically review all diabetic patients in the clinic, acting as an online consultant to all our primary care providers. I communicate with many patients through our EMR and have asked if I could start seeing my patients on video in their homes, but I was refused.

Future focus of activity: I want to use telemedicine with patients at home and set up monitoring systems for their blood sugars and vitals using apps and mobile devices so that I can work more asynchronously and with larger groups of patients. I want to make access better for my patients.

2. Teaching

Year in review: I have continuously run teaching sessions on endocrinology for all other providers at the clinic and have had good evaluations.

Future focus of activity: I would like to take part in the Project Echo grand rounds on diabetes that are soon to be available. This will increase my expertise and also allow me to contribute cases to the group.

3. Research and Creative Activities

Year in review: I have done very little research in the past year, mainly because I have not had enough extra time.

Future focus of activity: I want to evaluate and write up my internal e-consults on diabetes but need time and writing and statistical expertise to do this.

4. Service

Year in review: I have contributed to the clinic advisory committee of which I am a member and have continuously supported the change goals being set by our medical director.

Future focus of activity: I want to be able to take up more of a leadership position and start to use technologies more in the clinic to both improve patient care and increase our morale.

5. Self-Development

Year in review: My e-consult project has been a revelation to me. Not only do I really enjoy doing the consults, which I find very interesting and meaningful even if it means working asynchronously with patients, but I also like the peace and relaxation I can have while I am doing them, such as playing music in the background. I look forward to these sessions almost like a break. I have noticed that I have been able to think better and work out ways of managing the EMR much more efficiently as a result. I believe I have effectively become a super-user of the EMR.

Future focus of activity: I believe that more flexibility in my work would be great. I would like to be able to do 8 hours per week of my clinical asynchronous patient work at home, at times I choose, and move to a 4-day clinic week so I can more easily take long weekends to visit my family or enjoy myself. I think that using more technologies in my practice will be good for my patients, myself, and the clinic, and I would like to experiment with a range of these.

Planned Optimal Distribution of Effort Next Year

Ideally, I would like to spend at most 50% of my time in clinic but with a focus on becoming more efficient, doing more consults by telemedicine and by introducing apps and how they collect data to patients on a routine basis. I would like to increase my e-consults and asynchronous care to 30%, which will give me more time to evaluate these and write up the results. The other 20% of my time I would like to devote to managing introduction of Project Echo to the clinic and to teaching, mentoring, and supporting other physicians, with the goal of having them learn how to tame the EMR and use a variety of technologies with their patients so they, too, can become more efficient and in control of their work.

Lindy sat back and, after correcting a couple of minor typos, smiled and printed out two copies, one each for herself and Dr. Shaper. She knew that he would not allow her to do all that she wanted. He was just too conservative, and she was too radical, young, and different. But Lindy had been doing a lot of reading about how using technologies could actually prevent burnout and stress by making work more efficient, and she had decided she would talk with him about this in her mentoring sessions. After all, she thought, if my mom can connect with me on video just like all my friends, why am I not doing that with patients?

She walked from her room to meet with Dr. Shaper, feeling slightly nervous and worried that he might be more intrusive than she wanted in his attempts to get to know her and help advise her. As she took a seat in his office, she decided to start the conversation with a discussion around a difficult patient who was being poorly managed by one of the senior physicians in the clinic. Dr. Shaper gave her good advice about how to approach their colleague, having known him for the past 10 years. When they moved on to her research project and Dr. Shaper refused to give her extra time for it—while at the same time encouraging her to do it and offering to connect her with experts who could help—she became more hesitant, and by the time he asked to see her IDP, she felt sure she was overreaching in her requests for the coming year. She handed him a copy with great reluctance and sat back to await his reaction.

Dr. Shaper looked up thoughtfully. "This is really very interesting, Lindy. You seem to be wanting to make some quite radical changes in the way you work, certainly more than we've discussed in past sessions. Why is this? And you mention 'Project Echo,' which I've heard about but really don't understand well. What is Project Echo, and how could it help the clinic and our patients?"

Encouraged by this response, Lindy decided to jump in with both feet and explain her IDP proposal in full.

"Well, after beginning my e-consult project and being surprised at how effective it has been and how much I really enjoy it, I decided to do some research on how other technological approaches could be used to improve patient care and reduce physician burnout by making our work more meaningful and less stressful. I really want to work better than at present, and it seems to me that one of the approaches we could use at the clinic would be to greatly increase our use of technology with patients. After all, if I can talk to my family using video on my phone, which even my mom—who is phobic about computers—can do, why shouldn't I do the same with patients? For my generation, this is completely natural, and it has always seemed odd to me that we don't use internet-based technologies more for clinical care, as we do in our social lives. I decided I wanted to change how I work, and I thought this might be something I could lead at the clinic—hence my IDP requesting time to work on these issues. I spent quite a while searching online and learned about the American Telemedicine Association. I don't know if you are aware of this organization, but it's been around for 25 years and has about 10,000 members, including more than 400 companies and health systems. After exploring their website and downloading some of their clinical guidelines, I also managed to speak to several members. They're doing amazing things, many with the intention of providing better-quality care than is currently available using traditional in-person techniques. I concluded that if I could use a variety of technologies such as videoconferencing, e-mail, and monitoring applications on smartphones, I could work much more smartly than I do now and start seeing and treating a larger panel of patients more effectively using synchronous and asynchronous consults. This is really just an extension of my current e-consults."

Lindy saw that Dr. Shaper was listening intently, seemingly fascinated. She continued.

"You asked about Project Echo. This is one of the tools that's commonly used to help educate providers on specific topics, such as diabetes. What happens is really just a series of virtual grand rounds presented either by experts in an academic medical center or by colleagues in other nonacademic clinics like ours. It started with trying to increase knowledge about hepatitis C and then expanded into all sorts of areas, such as opiate addiction and diabetes, all of which are key to the clinic needs. I think if I could get relevant clinicians at the clinic involved in these 'echo' sessions, we might significantly improve the level of care we provide. Of course, that would not happen overnight and would take a lot of organizing, so you can see from my IDP document that what I would really like to do is to take a leadership role in the clinic to implement the use of new communications technologies as widely as possible. That's really what I'm suggesting in my IDP."

Dr. Shaper decided he had to ask a few questions at this stage, but he thought he should be careful because he did not want to put Lindy off. He was delighted at the initiative she had shown and the breadth of her goals and was actually quite impressed at what she was saying. His immediate reaction internally was positive, especially because this was an area that he knew the clinic would have to work on but that he, personally, was not very technically savvy and did not feel confident in taking a lead. Plus, it was impossible for him to do everything—as his wife frequently reminded him—and he suddenly realized that this might be a great opportunity both to ensure that Dr. Isla stayed at the clinic, where she was valued, and at the same time to move forward on a whole new change agenda. He tried to keep his tone as positive and encouraging as possible.

"Lindy, this does sound really interesting, and my immediate response is positive. Tell me, have you, at a practical level, thought through a series of steps that might be necessary to start this process? How would you get going?"

"Well, first of all, I know I need to learn more about the possibilities and the evidence base for using the various communications technologies with patients. To do that, I would like to join the American Telemedicine Association and go to their next annual conference. Once I'm a member, I'll have access via their various membership groups to numerous people with the same interests—people who want to provide better-value care using technology. I'm hoping to connect with other internists around the state and the country and learn from them what works best and how to implement virtual care technologies, both for myself and across the clinic. This seems to be a huge opportunity to have many of our patients with complicated illnesses monitored at home or through apps so that we could prevent them from getting sick instead of always having to treat them after they are symptomatic. I guess it might be possible for me to visit other clinics where this has already happened, and a lot of journal articles and several books have been published that should help. So, the first practical step is to do a lot more self-education and then to take that and write a proposal for you and the clinic advisory committee to see how we might implement and fund whatever seems best."

"You have certainly thought this through, Lindy." Dr. Shaper interjected.

Lindy nodded, her excitement increasing. "Of course, in my IDP I have also talked about implementing Project Echo and helping all of our clinicians manage the EMR better. That's really why I'm asking to have 50% of my time for the next year to do this sort of work. One of the side effects I hope to see is a gradual reduction in burnout scores across the clinic. I recall that you ran burnout surveys about 6 months ago, and we were in line with most other similar clinics, with about 50% of the clinicians having at least one of the major symptoms of burnout. As far as I know, no studies have been done that directly connect improved telemedicine technologies in patient care with reduced burnout, although some anecdotal reports of this can be found in the literature. It seems to me that this could be a much more interesting study and broader than just looking at my e-consults. Why, we could use the clinic as a pilot site to see if improved workflow and efficiency mediated by technologies is really associated with reduced burnout scores! That would be fascinating and is really where my passion lies." Lindy looked up hopefully and met Dr. Shaper's eyes. "What do you think?"

"I have to say, you have a tremendous vision, Lindy. All that you say makes sense, but I wonder how you thought to link technology innovations with burnout? They don't seem naturally connected to me."

"Actually, I respectfully disagree with you, Jack. Maybe it's partly my generation versus yours. As you know, my whole social world is connected through technologies. I couldn't survive without the internet. I really enjoy meeting my friends in person and socializing, but I keep up with them online constantly. I have personally found this really helpful since I moved here from the East Coast, where all my lifelong friends and family live. We are in constant electronic contact, and we see each other in person when I go back. It's just natural to me, and I don't see why we shouldn't be applying the same principles to patients as we do to our friends and family. We know that keeping connected in our social lives is good for our mental health, so why shouldn't keeping connected in multiple fashions also be good for our health at work if it allows us to have better and more flexible doctor–patient relationships? It all just seems logical to me and is something I've been discussing with several of my physician friends from residency who feel the same way. I guess what I'm asking you for is a chance to see if we can implement some of these technologies within the clinic and let them become part of routine patient care."

Dr. Shaper stroked his chin thoughtfully. "You've given me a great deal to think about, Lindy. What you say makes a lot of sense, and I detect a combination of passion, as you say, but also some frustration in your tone. You seem to want to make a lot of changes, perhaps more than other members of the clinic would be comfortable with, but I recognize that what you're talking about is inevitable, and the endpoint is not really something we should be debating. It's really about how do we get there, and can you be the driver of this sort of clinic-wide change?"

Lindy was happy and encouraged by his positive reaction. "I really appreciate you listening to me today, Jack. And I'm very grateful for your openness on this issue."

Dr. Shaper looked at his watch and started to conclude the session. "I'll tell you what, Lindy. I'll spend some time on the American Telemedicine Association website doing my own research. If you could send me a couple of papers to read that you think are good guides for how these technologies can be introduced, I'd appreciate it. Then we can discuss this further at our next session. I wonder if you could be a bit more specific when you rewrite the next version of your IDP about this topic and include something on the possible reduced burnout levels in the clinic as one of the outcomes."

"Sure. Thanks, Jack. I will certainly do that. It's been good seeing you today." She got up from her chair and left the room, pleased and feeling much more positive about her future, even thinking she might consider staying at the clinic if she could be given such an interesting role, despite Nana's health problems.

Lindy went to her office and sat at her desk to catch up on her inbox, but she quickly found she just couldn't concentrate; she was still quite excited about her session with Dr. Shaper. She had never felt this way in any of the previous sessions she had had with him, but she felt that this time he had really listened to her, and his responses had validated the importance and the positive aspects of the social and generational differences between them. She decided to phone her best friend from residency, Stacie, also an African American internist, who was married and had two young children. Stacie had stayed on the East Coast; Lindy knew she worked part-time from home for a telemedicine company helping to manage an inpatient geriatric unit several states away. Stacie had been encouraging her to have this discussion with Dr. Shaper and had been the source of much of the information that she had given to him.

"Hi Stacie. How are you?"

"I'm good, Lindy. Wasn't today the day you were putting forward your plan to your supervisor?"

"It sure was. Before I get to that, how are Janae and Silvia? If we switch to video, can you put them on?"

"You know, you are so out of touch with parenting and time zones, Lindy," Stacie answered. "My girls are at preschool right now. In fact, you're lucky to catch me; I've just been dealing with a sweet old lady with early dementia who keeps trying to leave the inpatient unit I manage. She has no idea where she is and just wants her son to take her out for dinner. She keeps looking for him. Anyway, I was just meeting with the nurses on video to work out a plan for her. Enough of that; tell me how it went!"

"Well, it went great. We had the best conversation we've ever had. Dr. Shaper really seemed to be listening to me, and more importantly, I felt truly respected. He was interested in all the virtual-care ideas, and it was nice to know so much more about a topic than he did. And he seemed fine about that, so I didn't feel the same gap between us that I have in the past. I even made the point you suggested about how you and I socialize online and in person, and why shouldn't we do that with patients? He seemed to get that, in particular. You know, this is one of the first times I haven't felt like a young junior female in his presence. I wasn't intimidated at all today, and I wasn't worried about how he saw me. He's always been friendly and warm, but today I felt I suddenly gained a great deal of respect from him that I haven't felt in the past. I felt like I was being treated like the medical specialist I am. Anyway, whatever the cause, whether it's my fault or his, it doesn't really matter. The key thing is that he said he would consider what I was saying and even asked me to give him some more information that I thought would be helpful for him."

"That's great. Well done. Sounds like the session went really well," Stacie commented.

"It did, and I feel so much more confident and optimistic about the future. You know, I may even stay at the clinic if he lets me do what I've proposed. Thank you for telling me how much you like seeing patients on video and working more flexibly from home; I made exactly that point to Dr. Shaper and said that introducing these new ways of working may well reduce burnout through the clinic. He really sat up when I said that, and he asked me to specifically put that into my IDP as an outcome. It's interesting. He really is concerned not just for patients but for his staff as well, and the point about using technologies to reduce burnout seemed to really hit a target with him."

Commentary

I explore two important issues in this chapter, both of which reduce the risk of burnout and are gradually being introduced throughout medicine. The first, following on from Chapter 3, is mentorship, which I have depicted from both mentor and mentee perspectives, including an examination of the concept of implicit bias and how it can often adversely affect the outcomes of the relationship, as is likely the case for both characters in this scenario. As part of the mentoring relationship, formal career planning is discussed, something that seldom happened for physicians in the early stages of their careers in the past but that is now becoming much more common. As such, I described Lindy's creation of her IDP and showed how it can be used to help her career decisions. The second issue is the importance of working more efficiently, one of the core components of the Stanford Wellness Program (Stanford Medical Center 2017), but in Lindy's case, this involves using information technologies such as the EMR and telemedicine more effectively. This approach is in contrast to most of the current medical literature, which focuses mainly on the unintended consequences of technologies, especially EMRs, in causing burnout by increasing administrative time and reducing patient-facing time for most physicians (Sinsky et al. 2016). Lindy also is determined to make her work more interesting and less stressful by using a series of innovative techniques, such as telemedicine, mobile devices, and apps, that she knows would make her work more enjoyable as well as more flexible, giving her more time with patients (Yellowlees and Shore 2018).

Increasing numbers of papers and reports on mentoring are becoming available, although little formal research and few scientific studies have been published, so most of the evidence in support of mentoring as an effective career tool is anecdotal, with evidence coming primarily from personal experiences. Among the many associations and groups encouraging and supporting mentoring relationships Lindy could have joined is the American Medical Women's Association (www.amwa-doc.org), which has impressive resources about mentoring on its website, in particular a series of important tips for continuously improving mentoring relationships. These tips, which would have helped both Dr. Shaper and Dr. Isla, appear in Tables 4–1 and 4–2 and are a good guide for both mentors and mentees.

The most recent systematic review of the process and outcomes of mentoring (Kashiwagi et al. 2013) focused on academic physicians. In this group, the authors identified seven mentoring models: dyad, peer, facilitated peer, speed, functional, group, and distance, of which the dyad model, as seen with Dr. Shaper and Dr. Isla, was most common. Seven components of a formal mentoring program were also identified: mentor preparation, planning committees, mentor-mentee contracts, mentor-mentee pairing, mentoring activities, formal curricula, and program funding. Kashiwagi et al. (2013) noted that written agreements were important to set limits and encourage accountability to the mentoring relationship, as the IDP in the scenario did. Rather sadly, they concluded that program evaluation was mainly subjective, with no programs that they found reporting long-term results or outcomes. Clearly, a need exists for considerably more scientifically focused research on mentoring.

What else do we know about mentoring that might have helped Dr. Shaper and Dr. Isla, who both seemed motivated to continue the rela-

---

TABLE 4–1. **Tips for mentors**

---

1. **Understand personal desires**

   Get to know your mentees on an individual and personal level and learn about their hopes, dreams, and goals beyond their current career decisions.

2. **Acknowledge conflicts of interest**

   Assess whether a conflict of interest or an emotional connection exists that will influence your guidance; if so, find them a mentor better suited to their needs.

3. **Ask open questions**

   Ask open questions and allow mentees to speak freely about their needs, values, and passions.

4. **Act as a sounding board**

   Be a good listener and allow mentees to share their concerns with you.

5. **Provide a fresh perspective**

   Provide your mentees with a fresh perspective on an issue, perhaps from your own experience.

6. **Seek out new experiences**

   Take the time to find and offer opportunities to your mentees, such as job opportunities, speaking engagements, research opportunities, scholarships or grants, and leadership opportunities.

7. **Choose feedback carefully**

   Not all feedback is helpful.

8. **Build confidence**

   Build your mentees' confidence by acknowledging their achievements and celebrating their successes.

9. **Share personal obstacles**

   Be comfortable sharing your own mistakes and failures.

10. **Offer advice when asked**

    Be a sounding board and, if asked, provide advice.

Source. Adapted from American Medical Women's Association 2012b.

tionship and who both had fairly similar goals for their workplace? Straus et al. (2013) described, in a study of 54 faculty members, that successful mentoring relationships were characterized by reciprocity, mutual respect, clear expectations, personal connection, and shared values. On the other hand, they concluded that failed mentoring relationships were characterized by poor communication, lack of commitment, personality differences, perceived (or real) competition, conflicts of interest, and the mentor's lack of experience.

From what we know of the relationship between Dr. Isla and Dr. Shaper, both partners could have been helped by improving their com-

TABLE 4–2.　Tips for mentees

1. Clarify your goals for mentoring. Why do you want a mentor? Define what type of help you are looking for in a mentor.
2. Determine how to find a specific mentor who matches your particular goal. Examine your personal network to identify potential mentors for reaching your goal.
3. Establish goals for the relationship. Discuss the goals of the relationship and whether or not the mentor is comfortable helping you achieve those goals. Create a development plan with your mentor.
4. Find more than one mentor. Seek out additional mentors who can advise you in a variety of situations. Also, consider peer mentors and individuals navigating the same life decisions at the same time you are.
5. Establish communication methods and frequency of contact. Determine how to communicate—in person, e-mail, video, or phone.
6. Manage expectations. Be realistic about what you expect to receive from your mentoring relationship.
7. Be respectful. Mentoring takes time. Do not overburden your mentors.
8. Do your part. Keep your appointments and follow through on leads and contacts they have provided to you.
9. Express your gratitude. Be sure the relationship is mutually beneficial and think of ways in which you can give back to them.
10. Explore a variety of mentoring options such as attending meetings and conferences and discussing written materials, including your resume or articles you have written.
11. Reevaluate your goals at scheduled intervals. Over time, your desires may change.

Source.　Adapted from American Medical Women's Association 2012a.

munication, because although they superficially have a reasonable working relationship, it clearly was not especially honest or open on either side. Dr. Shaper was trying to explore Dr. Isla's personal and career desires but was unable to do so in any detail, making him feel somewhat intimidated and uncertain. He had always found making new relationships difficult and tended to use formality, as might a "central casting physician," as a defensive style. As a consequence, he did not have the skills or knowledge to be more transparent with Dr. Isla during their conversations. Similarly, Dr. Isla did not feel comfortable enough with him to share her hopes, dreams, and goals because she also seemed to have some inherent personal biases and uncertainties leading to her defensiveness and lack of openness. These were likely related to prior negative or racist experiences as a black professional female interacting with older white males. She thus lacked the capacity to take a risk and open up so she could benefit as much from this relationship as she had from prior mentoring experiences during her residency.

It is logical to assume that both Dr. Shaper and Dr. Isla also each had their own implicit biases, which may have been part of the reason their mentoring relationship was not as strong as it might have been. *Implicit biases* are thoughts and feelings that tend to exist outside of conscious awareness and thus are difficult to consciously acknowledge and control. They are often automatically activated and can influence human behavior without conscious volition. In the United States, as Hall et al. (2015) identified in their systematic review of the topic, people of color face disparities in access to health care, the quality of care received, and health outcomes partly due to the implicit attitudes and behaviors of health care providers. In their review of 15 studies, low to moderate levels of implicit racial/ethnic bias were found among health care professionals in all but one study. They reported that these implicit bias scores against black, Hispanic/Latinx, and dark-skinned people were similar to those in the general population and that implicit bias in health care was significantly related to patient–provider interactions, treatment decisions, treatment adherence, and patient health outcomes. A more recent systematic review by FitzGerald and Hurst (2017) came to similar conclusions. This is clearly another area that merits much more study and one that health care professionals need to be aware of in their relationships with their colleagues and their patients.

Moving now to the second major component of this scenario, one that is a recurring theme throughout this book: How is it that health technologies can actually increase efficiency and potentially reduce burnout levels, as Dr. Isla proposed?

Study after study has demonstrated that the EMR is one of the current prime causes of burnout and physician distress, with a recent high-profile study (Sinsky et al. 2016) reporting that physicians spent 2 hours on the EMR and paperwork for every 1 hour with patients during their working day, and another average of 1.5 hours per day after office hours. The interaction of the EMR and its association as a cause of burnout is well described and was recently reviewed (Yellowlees 2018), so the issue for most physicians nowadays, and for Dr. Isla and Dr. Shaper, is not only how to tame the EMR and have it work for rather than control them but also how to integrate it into an efficient workflow that puts patient care first. Most health systems are working on how to make EMR documentation more efficient and less time consuming for all clinicians. Several also are focusing on attempts to reduce the volume of documentation that U.S. physicians write. This follows a fascinating recent comparison of the length of medical record consultations that showed that U.S. physicians commonly write up to three times more characters per ambulatory note than European or Australian doctors, with no discernible benefit and mainly driven by billing and administrative requirements (Downing et al. 2019). A range of approaches has been tried to speed up documentation, including the use of templates, scribes, dictation, and dictation software as well as various fixed and mobile hardware devices, such as laptops, tablets, dedicated data entry devices, and smartphones. The task for all physicians is to work out what suits them best in their environment so that they can be as efficient as possible and create good-quality professional notes that ideally are finished by the time the patient leaves the room, as was the case when notes were handwritten during the patient consultation.

Dr. Isla, however, has discovered from her exploration of telemedicine that working with patients on video can be much less stressful than seeing patients in clinic. She has learned about "hybrid" doctors, described by Yellowlees and Shore (2018), who see patients both in person and online, depending on mutual choice and convenience, and use technology to stay well themselves. Figure 4–1, which also appeared in Yellowlees and Shore (2018), is a brief summary of how to use technologies with patients in a way that is efficient but clinically appropriate and that saves time and stress for the physician.

Why is working with patients on telemedicine less stressful and likely better for physicians' overall health and well-being? Numerous reasons exist for the high satisfaction levels many physicians have with using telemedicine to see patients, as Stacie reported to Lindy. Discussed at length in Yellowlees and Shore (2018), they may be summarized as follows:

1. *Increased variety of work.* Seeing patients who are located in different places; seeing different types of patients by diagnosis, culture, or demographic status; or simply seeing some patients both in person and online increases the variety of the workday, making it less repetitive.
2. *Increased time with patients.* Surprisingly, perhaps, it is becoming clear that seeing patients on video actually gives doctors more time to spend with them per consultation, on average. Doctors frequently find two big time savers when using telemedicine. First, it is much easier to type up notes while talking to the patient, because in the telemedicine consultation it is possible to maintain good eye contact while using two or more screens simultaneously to type notes out of sight of the patient, with little interference in the relationship. Sec-

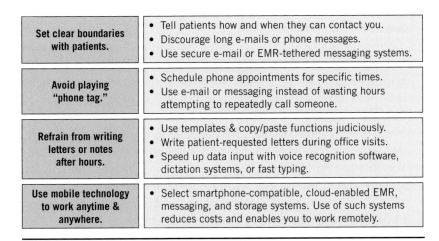

Set clear boundaries with patients.	• Tell patients how and when they can contact you. • Discourage long e-mails or phone messages. • Use secure e-mail or EMR-tethered messaging systems.
Avoid playing "phone tag."	• Schedule phone appointments for specific times. • Use e-mail or messaging instead of wasting hours attempting to repeatedly call someone.
Refrain from writing letters or notes after hours.	• Use templates & copy/paste functions judiciously. • Write patient-requested letters during office visits. • Speed up data input with voice recognition software, dictation systems, or fast typing.
Use mobile technology to work anytime & anywhere.	• Select smartphone-compatible, cloud-enabled EMR, messaging, and storage systems. Use of such systems reduces costs and enables you to work remotely.

FIGURE 4–1. **How to use technology to stay sane.**

EMR=electronic medical record.

Source. Diagram by Steven Chan, M.D., M.B.A. Used with permission.

ond, less time is spent rooming patients than in the physical office because patients are usually already lined up in a clinic or at home and are ready to be seen; they do not have to be settled into a clinic environment. These two differences can save 3–5 minutes per patient consultation. Given today's expectations of 15- to 30-minute consultations, this can make a substantial difference and allow a physician to hurry less and get to know the patient better.

3. *Increased collaboration and teamwork.* It is common to use telemedicine to see patients who are with a primary care provider in another clinic or to have experts such as psychiatrists beamed in to work with a clinic's primary care physician. Such collaboration helps patients directly and teaches and supports primary care providers.

4. *Increased flexibility of hours.* Patients can be seen literally anytime, anywhere and are no longer tied to the typical 8 A.M.–5 P.M. clinic day. Evening and weekend clinics suddenly become an option, and these may be much more convenient for both patients and physicians. Doctors thus may work from home and take time off during the day midweek if they wish. Part-time work is a popular option that is not offered in many traditional health systems or clinics but that young physician mothers, or more senior physicians, may greatly prefer.

5. *Increased flexibility and reduced cost of office environment.* Many physicians prefer working from home, where they can simultaneously, for

instance, look after their children, save travel time, and reduce the costs of an office by not having to rent rooms and pay support staff.

6. *Capacity to develop specialized clinical expertise.* A physician who likes looking after inpatients may be able to work in several hospitals simultaneously, whereas another who enjoys forensic work can attend more jails or prisons than would be possible in person.

7. *Increased safety.* Much has been written about the unfortunate fact of life that in certain specialties, such as emergency medicine, orthopedics, pain management, and psychiatry, some patients can be quite threatening. When seeing these patients via telemedicine, the distance involved indubitably enables the physician to feel physically safer. This has been noted many times in relation to female forensic physicians in particular.

Many of these work advantages can be gained within a clinic situation such as described in the scenario if management is supportive, as it seems Dr. Shaper is likely to be, and there is a "clinical champion," which is exactly the role Dr. Isla is proposing for herself. In this role, she would spend a proportion of her time exploring clinical innovations and teaching others in the clinic how to implement them successfully.

Dr. Isla is already doing a series of e-consults through the EMR, which she enjoys. Next, she might want to consider expanding these asynchronous consultations over time, perhaps going directly to patients or setting up access to other physicians who are not available within the clinic, such as dermatologists and ophthalmologists, or to cardiologists and gastroenterologists perhaps within the clinic, to do as she is doing by helping manage panels of patients. This easier access to subspecialty physicians will likely make the work of all the general clinicians easier and consequently less stressful.

Dr. Isla also mentioned joining echo virtual grand rounds to increase the knowledge of the primary care providers in the clinic (University of New Mexico School of Medicine 2018), initially for diabetes but later for a range of other mainly chronic medical conditions. Project Echo is described as follows on its website:

> Project ECHO is a lifelong learning and guided practice model that revolutionizes medical education and exponentially increases workforce capacity to provide best-practice specialty care and reduce health disparities. The heart of the ECHO model is its hub-and-spoke knowledge-sharing networks, led by expert teams who use multi-point videoconferencing to conduct virtual clinics with community providers. In this way, primary care doctors, nurses, and other clinicians learn to provide excellent specialty care to patients in their own communities.

　　　　Having been started in 2003 by Dr. Arora, a New Mexico hepatitis
expert who started virtual grand rounds to educate primary care providers about hepatitis C, as of 2018 Project Echo operates more than 220
hub sites for more than 100 diseases and conditions in 31 countries and
is a tremendous training resource for clinics and primary care providers
worldwide. (University of New Mexico School of Medicine 2018)

In summary, opportunities for both Dr. Shaper and Dr. Isla are many.
Their mentoring relationship hopefully will improve over time as they
get to know each other better and overcome their mutual implicit biases.
Dr. Isla could take a leading role, supported by Dr. Shaper, in the use of
technology to improve patient care, with many potential gains from
their efforts—namely, patients with better access to improved quality
care; more knowledgeable, flexible, and autonomous providers; and,
from the clinic leadership perspective, improved staff morale and less
provider burnout and turnover. Dr. Shaper can pass on his knowledge
of leadership and change management and may be able to help Dr. Isla
develop into a physician leader of the future, one who understands the
importance of physician well-being.

References

American Medical Women's Association: Building Mentoring Relationships:
　　How to Improve Yourself Through Mentoring (website). Schaumburg, IL,
　　American Medical Women's Association, 2012a. Available at: https://
　　www.amwa-doc.org/building-mentoring-relationships-how-to-improve-
　　yourself-through-mentoring. Accessed September 21, 2019.
American Medical Women's Association: 10 Ways to Improve Your Mentoring
　　Relationship. Schaumburg, IL, American Medical Women's Association,
　　2012b. Available at: https://www.amwa-doc.org/news/10-ways-to-
　　improve-your-mentoring-relationship. Accessed September 21, 2019.
Downing NL, Bates DW, Longhurst CA: Physician burnout in the electronic
　　health record era. Ann Intern Med 170(3):216–217, 2019 30716744
FitzGerald C, Hurst S: Implicit bias in healthcare professionals: a systematic re-
　　view. BMC Med Ethics 18(1):19, 2017 28249596
Hall WJ, Chapman MV, Lee KM, et al: Implicit racial/ethnic bias among health
　　care professionals and its influence on health care outcomes: a systematic
　　review. Am J Public Health 105(12):e60–e76, 2015 26469668
Kashiwagi DT, Varkey P, Cook DA: Mentoring programs for physicians in aca-
　　demic medicine: a systematic review. Acad Med 88(7):1029–1037, 2013
　　23702518
Sinsky C, Colligan L, Li L, et al: Allocation of physician time in ambulatory prac-
　　tice: a time and motion study in 4 specialties. Ann Intern Med 165(11):753–
　　760, 2016 27595430

Stanford Medical Center: Stanford Wellness Framework. Well MD, Stanford Medicine (website), 2017. Available at: https://wellmd.stanford.edu. Accessed July 13, 2018.

Straus SE, Johnson MO, Marquez C, et al: Characteristics of successful and failed mentoring relationships: a qualitative study across two academic health centers. Acad Med 88(1):82–89, 2013 23165266

University of New Mexico School of Medicine: Project Echo (website). Albuquerque, NM, University of New Mexico, 2018. Available at: https://echo.unm.edu. Accessed August 20, 2018.

Yellowlees P: Physician Suicide: Cases and Commentaries. Washington, DC, American Psychiatric Association Publishing, 2018

Yellowlees P, Shore J: Telepsychiatry and Health Technologies: A Guide for Mental Health Professionals. Washington, DC, American Psychiatric Association Publishing, 2018

Chapter 5

PRE-MED: VULNERABILITY AND TRAUMA

Scenario

Mr. Howard surveyed his class of 20 high school seniors who were sitting at their desks attentively listening to him. They all looked so young. All were serious and had their laptops open, either to take notes from the upcoming talk or to do something more interesting online. They had asked him to set up this talk, and he had been happy to oblige.

"As we discussed last week, it is a great pleasure to have Luis Garcia here. Luis was a senior here just over 5 years ago, and next semester he's going to start medical school. He is living proof that all of you can succeed if you work hard and plan your careers carefully. He is someone who is committed to helping his community, and it is very kind of him to come here and tell you his story. I hope it will give you some ideas for yourselves and the confidence to push yourselves forward to success, just like he has." He looked around the room. "Before I invite Luis to speak, I want to tell you a brief story about him. I first taught Luis when he was a junior in my biology class. As many of you have done, we had to do some dissection of frogs to examine their anatomy. It was evident that Luis really hated doing that, mainly because he didn't like the idea of the frogs being sacrificed for his learning. I remember that he looked queasy, and I thought he was going to be sick, but he managed to get over that and did a great dissection. When I spoke to him after class about how he felt, he told me he'd been thinking of trying to become a veterinarian or a doctor, and he was worried about the reaction he'd had to the frog. We had several long chats about this issue, and eventually Luis started dropping by to speak to me about other academic ideas he had. This led to him deciding to study biology at college, with the aim of going into one of the health professions. I'm not sure he'll ever be a surgeon, but I do know that he is a caring and gentle person who will make a great physician and will comfort a great many people, whatever he does."

Turning to Luis, Mr. Howard laughed, reminiscing. "I don't know if you remember that class, Luis, but you really did look like you were going to be sick. I'm looking forward to finding out what sort of physician you become. Maybe you could include some of your long-term ambitions in your talk today. I'm fascinated to know how you are thinking now." He turned back to his class. "Students, please welcome Luis back to his old school, and let's listen to his advice as to how to get through college and into medical school. Do please take over now, Luis."

Luis, who had been standing just behind his mentor, moved forward to address the class. "Being back at school in Mr. Howard's classroom is really like a homecoming for me. Just so all of you know, if you don't already, Mr. Howard was incredibly helpful to me, and I will always be grateful for everything you did, sir." He looked across at his longtime academic mentor gratefully and smiled. Mr. Howard looked down, somewhat embarrassed but secretly pleased at the acknowledgment. He certainly was pleased at how well Luis had done so far in his career.

Luis continued. "When Mr. Howard asked me to come and talk to you, he asked if I would tell you my story and about how I managed to get into medical school. He said he really wanted me to tell you what I have learned about the process, and what I will need to do in the future to become a good physician and help my future patients. Of course, I don't know *all* of that yet. I haven't even started medical school, but I've been accepted. It's been really hard to get here, and I'm so glad to be at this point in my life. I spent a lot of time learning about what I can expect. I wanted to know about the life of a physician and how it is changing; what I will likely be faced with in the future; and what sorts of skills and knowledge I will need to develop in order to become a good doctor while at the same time having a full and happy life in general. Mr. Howard told me that you are all studying STEM[1] topics, and some of you are aiming to go to a college with a pre-med program so that you can eventually become doctors. It's great that you are thinking and planning ahead, because that is one of the skills every good doctor needs."

He looked around the room and could see that he had everyone's attention; no one seemed to be browsing the web or posting on social media. Just as he was feeling confident that he had the whole class with him, his phone—sitting on the desk beside him—beeped. A tweet with a photo of him addressing the class had been posted. *So much for keeping their full attention!* he thought. At least one of them was on social media.

Luis decided to ignore Twitter, muted his phone, and focused on the audience. He felt surprisingly confident about giving this talk after all of the public speaking practice he had had recently, and he decided to ask them all to put their phones away and on mute so that they weren't distracted for the next hour. He had prepared the outline of this talk carefully and had the main points easily available—ironically, on his phone's note application—in case he became anxious and forgot to talk about some of his experiences. He had thought about how to dress for this occasion so that he could not only connect with the group but also look more professional than he usually did; his usual worn jeans and baseball cap would not suffice. He was wearing light slacks and a collared shirt with his best brown leather shoes. Giving up his attempt to grow a beard, he also had shaved for today, and his reflection in the mirror this morning had looked more mature and manly than usual.

"First, I want to make it clear that I am fine with you asking any questions as we go along. Just put your hand up. Second, I'm going to try to keep this talk a bit mysterious by not telling you which medical school I'm going to attend until the very end. That way, I can talk more about what I learned without biasing you, in case you happen to know the school." He took a breath.

"Let me start at the beginning of my story. I was about 10 years old when I first thought of trying to become a doctor, and I got serious about it when I entered high school. Let me ask you this: How old were you when you started to think seriously about medicine as a career? Who was like me and thought about this before middle school?"

About half the hands in the room went up. Luis chose a redheaded student in the second row and asked her to tell the class how her story began. "My name is Ann," she said. "And I can remember dressing up as a doctor when I was about 5 or 6 years old. We had a lot of ill health

---

[1]STEM = science, technology, engineering, and mathematics.

in my home; Dad was constantly sick and in bed, and I was the eldest of four children, so Mom really depended on me to help her. He died of chronic liver disease just before I started high school. Most of my life up to that time had been focused on him. I remember telling him when I was about 8 that I would become a doctor so I could cure him, because he had told me several times that there was no cure for his illness. I haven't ever really thought of doing anything else and have already done several volunteer jobs during school holidays, such as assisting at local clinics, where I get to see doctors working. My family doctor knows what I want to do and has told me that if I can get into pre-med at college, he will let me shadow him. I'm really looking forward to that."

"Thanks Ann," Luis responded. "It sounds like you've certainly made up your mind. What do your mom and others in your family think of your plan?"

"They mostly think it's a good idea, although my grandma is concerned about the amount of work I do to make sure my grades are good, never mind the time I spend going to clinics after school. She keeps saying I should have more fun and do some sports or art. But I think that if I want to succeed in something like being a doctor, I will always have to work hard. If that means sacrificing some of my other activities for a while, then I think that would be worth it. After all, how can I ever become a liver doctor, and help cure the disease that killed my dad, if I don't work hard?"

Luis looked intently at Ann and then addressed the whole class. "I wonder what everyone else thinks of what Ann is doing? She certainly sounds very determined. Are you doing the same? How hard do you think you have to work to get into medical school? Should you give up your outside interests?"

A boy wearing scruffy clothes and long, unkempt hair who was sitting in the back row responded almost immediately. "We all know Ann. She answers every question first, just like she did with you. She always wants to get the best grades and is super focused on work. It's a disaster, and she thinks she has failed completely, if she doesn't get an A+. We all know about her dad and his illness, and the other problems she had at home as a child, because she talks about them a lot. Personally, I think she makes too much of them; we have all told her lots of times that if she really does want to go to medical school, she should try to do other things apart from work. Who wants to see a doctor who has no other interests in life, who doesn't go to concerts or hang out with friends at least a few days a week? I certainly wouldn't."

"That's just because I always do better than you in class, Simon. You're jealous, as usual. In case you don't know, I do listen to music. A lot. At home," Ann responded defensively.

"Now, now guys," Luis intervened. "Let's not get too judgmental. But that's actually a really important point, Simon, and something I learned when I started finding out about how to get admitted to medical school. Ann, I know you're trying to do the right thing, but I also have sympathy for Simon's view in this case, and I think he means to give you good advice. One of the areas admissions committees look at is a person's life experiences and breadth of knowledge, and they much prefer applicants who have broad backgrounds and who have succeeded in areas outside of medicine. They want to see if students have really done things and participated in projects, possibly showing leadership qualities rather than observing much of the time, although doing some shadowing is always good because it makes you sure of your career decision. I certainly did that early on."

Luis decided he was being drawn a bit off track by this conversation and moved to bring his talk back to his original plan.

"We've talked about three key things so far about medical school admission. First, many students make up their minds to go into health care very early, perhaps sometimes too early. Second, quite a few kids go into medicine partly because of their life experiences of illness as children or adolescents, rather like Ann. Third, although hard work and a strong focus on getting good grades is essential, it's best if this can be combined with other interests or experiences outside of the health care world, especially through leadership roles in almost any area. My big message to you all is that it *is* possible to overcome adversity and do well in life, and becoming a doctor is one way of doing this. The trick is learning to both work hard and play hard, and to enjoy both."

Luis relaxed and sat on the desk at the front of the class, facing the students, with his legs dangling free in front and his torso and head slightly above theirs, a position that allowed him to dominate the group. "Now, let me tell you my personal story, and you'll see how all of those issues have been important to me. I was like Ann in many respects. I came from a poor family, and my father died when I was very young. I had a really difficult childhood; my mother didn't cope well with my brother and me, so we really had to bring ourselves up, often feeling neglected and very alone. By the time I was about 8 years old, I had started taking on the role of the male head of the household. I was responsible for my brother and for helping my mom, whom I now believe must have been depressed for years. She drowned her sorrows drinking cheap wine, or vodka in a 'water bottle' that never left her side, and eating comfort food. I remember scavenging from the dumpsters behind the supermarket to get food that had been thrown out. We had to go on public assistance for several years, and we lived in an awful area of the city, where gangs and violence surrounded us. Despite this, our situation forced me to work hard at school, and I think that's what saved me. I felt responsible for my younger brother, so I did the best I could. Like Ann, I was the eldest in the family, and from an early age I learned the importance of eating right—mainly because my overweight mother with insulin-dependent diabetes didn't do so. She was always talking to us about the importance of nutrition, but we knew perfectly well that she survived on fast food most of the time, and we were well aware that she was drinking heavily.

"By the time I was a teenager, Mom had remarried, to a man she had met at Alcoholics Anonymous. The whole family became overly focused on food and diets, perhaps as another form of addiction instead of alcohol. I was a bright, young kid, so I started to read a lot about this topic to try to understand why Mom's diabetes was so badly out of control. I remember doing a school project on diabetes and learning why my mom just kept getting sicker all the time; she was eating all the wrong things. I couldn't get her to change, but at least I began to understand what was going on with her. I was just a sensitive kid who was trying to do his best to help."

Luis continued to describe the development of his fascination with biology during high school, and how Mr. Howard had taken a real interest in him and had both mentored and challenged him academically. He talked about how he had become serious about getting into medical school by the time he was a sophomore. At that stage, he was helping run health booths with the local public health department on the weekends and began to understand the connections between basic biological processes and a number of diseases. He learned how to take vitals and simple histories from people attending the booth, and because he continued his volunteering throughout his time at high school, he ended up doing some simple counseling to attendees and giving out relevant literature on obesity, diabetes, and excessive drinking.

Luis tried to move through this section of the talk quickly, because he knew the students were all past this stage and would be more interested in what they were likely to face next. He emphasized that he became a runner because that sport cost no money, unlike football with all its attendant gear; he could literally just sprint out the front door to escape his sometimes-toxic home environment whenever he had time. He described learning that he had been sponsored to go on a school trip to Asia the summer after his senior year, which had given him a real taste for travel and seeing other cultures. He never had learned who the sponsor was.

"What did you do when you went to college? How could you afford it, and how did you pick your courses there?" asked a well-dressed, rather intent Hispanic student.

"The first thing I did was join the pre-med student society. In fact, one of the reasons I went to City University was because they had a strong pre-med program and seemed to have a lot of students succeed in getting into medical or health care graduate programs. But before that, I must emphasize that I did a *lot* of planning and researching. Mr. Howard pointed me in the right direction many times. He told me how to find lots of scholarships for people like me. It's amazing what's available on the internet, and how all the medical schools have differing academic prerequisites that you have to meet. Later I'll give you a list of websites I've found useful."

He continued. "You mentioned picking courses. That is crucial, because you don't want to suddenly find that you need to do physics at the same time as you are taking the MCAT or are about to submit your medical school application in AMCAS. Do you all know those acronyms? If you want to work in health care, you are going to have to love acronyms! The Medical College Admissions Test, or MCAT, is the exam all intending medical students have to take, and the American Medical College Admission Service, or AMCAS, is the place you apply to for entry. Anyway, getting back to your question, my advice is to make sure you use your college advisors and, at the same time, start to identify possible medical schools as early as you can and check out their requirements for admission."

Another student put up her hand. "I know that all medical schools are different, so what sorts of things did you look for when you started researching them to see where might be best for you? After all, we're all different individuals and have different needs."

"I'm really pleased you asked that question," Luis replied. "I think you all should be trying to match your own needs with your ideal school. Your question leads to what I think was the most important reason behind my decision regarding school choice, and it all happened during my final year of college, when I went to a special lecture arranged by the college pre-med society."

Luis paused while he collected his thoughts and wondered how much personal exposure would be appropriate.

"Let me give you a bit of background. For the first time in my life, about 18 months ago, I was having a really hard time. My grades had slipped, and I felt miserable for several months for no obvious reason. I was seriously thinking of abandoning the idea of medicine and doing something both easier and less stressful. I doubted that I could get into medical school and just wasn't sure which schools might suit me best, despite doing a lot of research. A whole lot of things happened at once. My girlfriend of 2 years left me, saying I was no fun anymore because I worked too much. She was angry with me and made a whole lot of nasty posts on Facebook that were very embarrassing and have haunted me since. I've heard all sorts of stories about the importance of a good on-line media profile for medical school admission. Anyway, she did finally agree to delete them before my school interviews, much to my relief, because having done the interviews, I now *know* it's important to have a good online profile. You all need to be aware of that and not allow yourselves to be photographed doing things that might embarrass you later.

"Anyway, at the same time all this was going on, I pulled a knee ligament during a pickup game of basketball and had to stop running for several months. Then my mom, who had already gone blind from her poorly controlled diabetes, had a heart attack and died suddenly at home. All of these things meant I wasn't keeping up with my studies and was just feeling totally beaten." Luis looked around the room and could see that the students had not been expecting this section of the story. They were completely quiet. A pin dropping would have been like a drumroll in the silent room.

He went on. "Imagine my reaction when I found out that the topic of the keynote lecture for our pre-med society annual meeting was 'physician well-being.' I was certainly pretty down and upset, and at times quite depressed, even tearful. I was doubting my career choice, but suddenly, here is this lecture topic that really piqued my interest. Possibly a good omen."

Luis stood up and walked around the front of the class, stretching his legs and taking his time. He wanted to give the students a message that, to him, was of great importance.

"So, I went to the lecture. Rather reluctantly, to be honest, but hopeful and eager to learn something that I might relate to. It turned out to be a life-changing event for me. My eyes were completely opened to the possibilities of medicine. I started to feel positive about my career choice again, although Mr. Howard is right, I cannot imagine being a surgeon. I'm sure most of you have had special moments happen that have been very influential for you. This was mine."

Luis looked across at Mr. Howard, the only person in the room who knew what was coming. He sought reassurance, which he received via an encouraging smile and a slight nod of the head. He continued.

"There's one thing I didn't mention earlier, when I talked about my family background and why I was so interested in going into medicine. I told you about my mom's diabetes, and how I had such a hard child-hood. How she was not a good patient, eating the wrong foods and not exercising. One of the reasons I had to help her so much was because my dad had died when I was only 2 years old, and I don't think my mom ever recovered from that. I found out years ago that my dad had been a doctor, although Mom always refused to talk about him. One of my reasons for being so keen on a medical career was to follow in his foot-steps." He paused. "What I had no idea about, until last year just before my mom died when she finally decided to tell me about him, was that he had had alcoholism and had eventually committed suicide. She had kept this a secret from the whole family all these years because of the stigma surrounding his death. A medical friend of his wrote 'cardiac ar-rest' on his death certificate, and everything was hushed up. The only reason Mom told me about this before she died was because she was afraid that if I went into medicine, I would do the same."

Luis stopped talking and momentarily looked out of the window. White puffs of clouds skated across a bright blue sky. The listening stu-dents were tense, surprised, and fascinated.

"She'd kept the suicide note he had written all those years ago and gave it to me a week before she died. It seems that he took a massive overdose of narcotic painkillers with whiskey and never woke up. His letter was so sad. He seems to have been overworking as the only family medicine doctor in the country town where we lived; he was always on call and always available. He described how he blamed himself for the death of a child because he believed he'd missed some early signs of meningitis, although my mom said that was not true. After that, he gradually lost confidence in his ability. In his letter to Mom, he said he felt hopeless, guilty, alone, and ashamed and didn't want any help, nor did he deserve it. He wrote that he was afraid that his 'mistake' would always be remembered by the community; that he would be unable to bear the public shame and blame; and that everyone would be better off without him. Mom said she had been trying to persuade him to see a colleague for help, but he kept refusing to the end, saying that all doctors were trained to be tough and to look after themselves."

Somewhat surprised by how painful this public discussion was, Luis took a moment of reflection, looking around at the students and meeting Mr. Howard's warm and friendly eyes. He held his emotions back with difficulty, although he could feel his tears forming, and pulled out a tissue to wipe his nose and eyes.

"You can imagine how painful it was to have suddenly discovered all this about my dad, while already having uncertainties about my own future. It was hardly surprising I was having doubts about my career choice. Going to that talk at that time was the best thing I could have ever done, because it made me think of medicine in a different light. The speaker acknowledged that even doctors were humans and had problems, but she was really hopeful and optimistic about the ways they could be helped. I'd been thinking that with all my family problems I would not be able to manage medical school, but I suddenly now saw that this was possible and that many schools had extra help available for students who were having difficulties. Why, the lecturer even talked about how helping doctors was becoming a new potential career path for some physicians—a bit like being a car mechanic preventing cars from deteriorating, if you see what I mean."

A hand went up, rather hesitantly, belonging to a young black student. "I don't quite get it," he said. "How can that be a career path? Was she talking about her own experiences? And why would you want to work in that area after what happened to your dad?"

"You're right to ask those questions," Luis responded. "I must say that when I went to the talk, I was expecting that the speaker, who was a family physician like my dad, would be talking about her own experiences or something like that. But I was completely wrong. She did talk a lot about the stresses of practicing medicine and how, over the years, she has changed her practice. She now specializes in seeing physicians and has many doctors as patients in her half-time clinical practice. She said she has much more control over how she practices, and her patients are all prepared to pay for her to spend more time with them than used to be the case when she had a more general practice. She does all the regular medical checkups they need, and she works closely with a small network of psychiatrists, addiction specialists, and internal medicine experts to whom she can refer patients if necessary. She made the point that by doing that, she was not only providing better care for her patients but also practicing what she called 'self-care' because she found her new style of practice much less personally stressful."

Another student chimed in. "My name is Claire, and I'm planning on pre-med next year. I think I understand where you're going with this, but it's just so odd to think that doctors need help. They always seem to be the ones we go to for help. We just assume that doctors take care of themselves and do what they tell everyone else to do. I think of doctors as being so committed that they pretty much work all the time because that's just what they do. It's their job."

"Yes," Luis answered. "We all expect doctors to work hard, but they also need time to refresh, like everyone else. It's part of being healthy. The basics of good nutrition and work-life balance are critical for doctors. You can't be effective if you're worn out and not feeling your best. It actually takes thinking and planning to keep fit and healthy, and doctors must do that for themselves—not just tell everyone else to do it. Some articles now describe how to identify and treat doctors like my dad, and others who have addictions, as well as lots who were burned out, mainly from administrative demands. To me, the most important message is that all doctors need to focus on self-care much more. It made me really think about my dad. My mom swore that my dad was found not to be responsible for the death of that child. She said he'd become depressed and worn out, and the child's death was the final straw. He worked 12–14 hours a day and made rounds most weekends. He apparently had no outside interests. Doctors didn't really seek help in those days. Colleagues didn't intervene. It was just ignored, and that's what finally did it. He was tired and lost hope along the way." Luis stopped again. He thought deeply about how best to move on with his talk.

"I said that going to that talk was life changing for me, especially in relation to finding out about my dad. Well, it made me suddenly think that aiming to become a doctor in order to help other doctors, and maybe also other types of health care professionals, would be a really rewarding career. I can't be sure if that's what I will end up doing, of course, but at least it's an interesting option to think about and to explore. It made me think very differently about medical school and led me to do a lot more research on which school to go to."

Mr. Howard put up his hand. "Luis, you will have to finish in a few minutes. I wonder if you could focus on your research and how it led to you selecting possible medical schools for yourself?"

"Certainly. Thanks, Mr. Howard. Well, it was tricky. When you look at what most medical schools put on the internet for pre-med students, the topic of physician well-being really doesn't come up much at all. Hardly anything can be found on the subject, even on the AAMC— that's the Association of American Medical Colleges—website, which is really surprising to me. So, I went to my faculty mentor at City University, but she didn't really have many ideas. I remembered that Mr. Howard had always said I could come back to see him, so that's what I did. We spent an hour together searching for education programs on physician health, and I hate to think how much extra time you spent on your own, Mr. Howard, but the list of resources you sent me was great. The breakthrough came when Mr. Howard asked me if I'd followed up with the doctor who'd given the lecture on physician well-being. I felt like a complete fool, because she was the obvious person to approach! So that's what I did. She was kind enough to see me and was able to give me a whole lot of good inside knowledge about what sort of school to go to and which have the best well-being programs for students and faculty. Surprisingly, she told me no specific training programs have been established yet for doctors who want to treat or help doctors, although they are being developed and might be around by the time I'm through residency."

"What did she suggest you do then, Luis?" asked Mr. Howard.

"She was really practical and helpful. She said that I should first look for a medical school that has a strong wellness program and a lot of resources to help students, because that is a clear indicator that they see student health as being of great importance. Then she said to look for the ones that also seemed to have similar programs for residents, which again are usually straightforward to find and compare. Next, she suggested I check out the schools' interests in primary care and public health, and whether they were strong in these areas, and also determine if they had good residency programs in primary care and psychiatry, which she thought would be the most relevant disciplines. Her overall view was that if a medical school covered all of these bases, it would most likely provide me with training opportunities I would value. I did all of that. It's surprising how few medical schools exist that meet all of those criteria. I was able to search among my top medical schools and pick out the ones that seemed to have the best programs, and those were the schools I listed as my top preferences. Then, when I was lucky enough to be offered four interviews, I made sure that I asked about wellness as much as possible when I visited the schools, to gauge how effective the programs were and what level of commitment they really had to them."

Another hand went up from a woman in the back row. "Still, it must be hard to try and work out the best school when there really aren't any training programs in the field you think you want to work in. Did you do anything else?"

"Good point," said Luis. "I guess I was lucky. Dr. Evansly, the well-being lecturer, was just wonderful with me and was more than willing for me to contact her again and run my ideas past her. Of course, she had her own biases and made it clear that she thought I should apply to *her* medical school, which was one of the four that I interviewed with. I telephoned her after each interview to process what I'd learned, and she was amazingly helpful by both listening and gently challenging me. She pointed out that, although right now I'm primarily interested in physician well-being, medical students typically change their minds about long-term career choices several times during medical school, and she advised me to keep my eyes open for other options at all times. Anyway, despite that warning, which makes a lot of sense to me, the end result was that I accepted the offer of going to State University's medical school. That's where Dr. Evansly works, and as an add on, she has already volunteered to be one of my mentors and has shown me several possible scholarships I can apply for so I might have less student debt long term."

"That's great! Congratulations," said Claire. "It must be great to have such good contact with a faculty member before you even go to medical school. Do you have any other connections there already?"

"Actually, I do," Luis replied. "The school has a system of colleges, with about one-quarter of each year belonging to each of the four colleges, so when you start you have a built-in student support system that runs through all 4 years of the course. I've already had several students contact me from my college and have met a couple of them for coffee. They've given me the lowdown on what I need to do to prepare for the first year, and as a result, I'm already doing extra reading in biochemistry to prepare myself, because that's my weakest subject. I hope I'm not putting you guys off, but medical students still have to master the precise details of all the liver enzymes and the Krebs cycle to be a doctor. I guess one of my objectives for school could be to try to improve the curriculum so it includes useful topics that doctors have to know in order to practice, such as taking care of their own health. That would make the experience of medical school much more useful and relevant and would provide real-life tools to deal with stress and very hard work."

Luis looked around the room, ready to finish his talk. "You know, preparing this talk for you guys has been very helpful to me. I think I may look at doing some sort of review of what might make a good curriculum for anyone who wishes to be a 'doctor's doctor.' I think that would have made both my parents very proud. I wish they could have seen what I'm doing."

Commentary

Three major themes of this scenario are important. First, what strengths or evidence of resilience and motivation do schools look for in applicants that will ensure chosen students have long-term success as physicians? The corollary is what, therefore, do students have to demonstrate to obtain admission to medical school? A related issue is how can students carefully curate their online presence and their offline resume over several years to ensure that they minimize possible "red flags" that might obstruct their admission?

Second, what programs do medical schools have to support the well-being of their students? We know from the research of Brazeau et al. (2014) that, at entry to medical school, medical students are more resilient than age- and gender-matched nonmedical graduate students. Yet within 2 years they have higher rates of depression and burnout than equivalent control subjects, and these high rates persist throughout residency and for at least 5 years beyond (Dyrbye et al. 2014). What goes wrong, and how can this be prevented?

Third, despite Luis's obvious motivation and intelligence and his demonstrated capacity to overcome adversity, it is evident that he is someone who is vulnerable to becoming burned out or psychiatrically ill in the future. He may need extra support and help during his training as well as later on in his career. How do we know this? Luis has a strong genetic predisposition to depression, through his father's suicide, his mother's likely chronic depression (and diabetes as a second chronic illness), and his own possible recent episode of depression. Just as importantly, he has a background characterized by adverse childhood experiences (ACEs), which we know are related to an increased risk of poor mental and physical health outcomes in adulthood. Were he to take it, Luis would score more than 4 on the ACE Scale (Gilbert et al. 2015) as a consequence of his traumatic childhood. This cutoff score is associated strongly with the likelihood of the eventual development of chronic medical and psychiatric disorders in adulthood. In summary, Luis is vulnerable both biologically or genetically and from a lifestyle and experiential perspective. What are the implications of this for his future career as a physician despite his capacity to successfully jump the high bars related to medical school admission?

Taking the first theme in this chapter, what do medical schools look for in applicants that, they believe, will create successful doctors? Luis learned the importance of self-care and well-being years before entry to medical school but, during the entry process, also discovered how relatively little medical schools, residencies, and postgraduate academic programs focus currently on this topic. Medical schools' admissions teams use many differing data points to help them predict which students will cope well with the ardors of medical school and residency training and become successful physicians and which will not. These include not only students' performances on the MCAT and their grade point averages in college but also their capacity for self-care and resilience, which, although often demonstrated by students, is harder to objectively measure. At a broader level, it is well known that doctors need to be both caring and organized to succeed professionally. As a result, medical school admissions committees frequently look for personality characteristics in students that show evidence of some dependency and compulsiveness, both traits that unfortunately can make the individuals vulnerable to developing psychiatric disorders if present to an excessive level. At the same time, they are looking to exclude students who have little empathy with, or sympathy for, other people.

Some interesting studies of the personalities of medical students examined these issues in more detail. A recent large study of 808 medical students at the University of Queensland, Australia, published by Eley et al. (2016) identified two distinct personality profiles. Profile 1 ("resilient") characterized 60% of the sample and was distinguished by low harm avoidance combined with very high persistence, self-directedness, and cooperativeness. Profile 2 ("conscientious") showed more harm avoidance and less persistence, self-directedness, and cooperativeness. The research team concluded that both profiles were indicative of mature and healthy personalities, but the combination of traits in Profile 1 was more strongly indicative of well-being and resilience.

So what do medical schools who have a demonstrated interest in helping students with their own self-care look for in prospective medical students, and what could Luis have told his audience if he had fully understood the perspective of most schools? Morris (2016) summarized five key attributes that lead to successful medical school entry:

1. Communication skills: Medicine is dependent upon the communication of ideas, concepts, and orders.

2. Presence: This trait is key when effectively speaking to colleagues and patients. Be present by focusing attention on the other individual when talking.
3. Critical thinking: This is integral as the physician assesses volumes of data to quickly form a working conclusion, using deductive reasoning and inferences based on knowledge and experience.
4. Compassion: Compassion is more than kindness and civility; it's authentic sympathy for self, patients, colleagues and co-workers irrespective of race, class, creed or personal behavior.
5. Resilience: This is what gets you through those moments when seemingly everything has gone wrong. For a successful career and life, discover healthy coping mechanisms that work best for you to perform optimally.

In all, developing character along with learning scientific and technical knowledge creates a well-informed and balanced physician.

Morris includes resilience and coping skills as a key characteristic of those who succeed in medical school entry, and this character component can be seen on an increasing number of medical school admissions pages. Allegheny College, a small liberal-arts college in Pennsylvania, gives detailed suggestions to its students as to how they can eventually obtain admission to medical schools, including the following quote about self-care as a key admission component:

Ability to care for yourself: Medical schools want students (and eventually doctors) who can take care of themselves. This means students who know how to relax in a healthy, responsible way. This means knowing your limits and knowing enough to seek help when you have reached them. This means maintaining a healthy life style—eating healthy meals, sleeping a reasonable number of hours, getting regular exercise, and having a social support system—family and friends who will listen and help when times are rough. (Allegheny College 2019)

At the other end of the admissions scale, Dr. David Hall, dean of admissions at The David Geffen School of Medicine at University of California, Los Angeles, considers experience primarily in four areas as described on their website (Hall 2017):

1. Medical environments. "Perhaps they've interacted with patients in a clinic, volunteered with a mobile health program or worked as scribes for emergency departments," suggests Dr. Hall. "Shadowing opportunities are helpful, but not enough. They should have an active role in these experiences."

TABLE 5–1. **Fifteen core competencies that demonstrate preparedness for medical school**

Preprofessional competencies	Thinking and reasoning competencies	Science competencies
Service orientation	Critical thinking	Living systems
Social skills	Quantitative reasoning	Human behavior
Cultural competence	Scientific inquiry	
Teamwork	Written communication	
Oral communication		
Ethical responsibility to self and others		
Reliability and dependability		
Resilience and adaptability		
Capacity for improvement		

Source. Association of American Medical Colleges Staff 2017. © 2019 Association of American Medical Colleges. Reproduced with permission. All rights reserved.

2. Community service. "We look for humanistic qualities in applicants, so activities that involve caring for others are important."
3. Research. "Clinical research is directly applicable to how we treat and manage patients. So familiarity with the principles of research is important."
4. Leadership. "We're looking for students who want to become leaders in academic, community, research and policy areas. Leadership experience could come from being mentors or teachers, officers in student organizations or research [principal investigators] or coauthors. Leadership takes different forms."

Studentdoctor.net, an extensively used nonprofit website founded in 1999 that aims to provide unbiased advice to medical students, described in 2017 how, although each medical school has its own process for reviewing candidates, many evaluate applicants using *holistic review*, described as a flexible, individualized way for admission committees to consider an applicant. Balanced consideration is given to experiences, attributes, and academic metrics, just as Luis was telling his students. The website notes that a number of medical schools have worked together to create a comprehensive list of 15 core competencies for prospective medical students (Table 5–1), with a strong focus on what are described as *preprofessional* competencies—the softer and harder-to-describe factors that contribute to self-care and resilience.

These broad core competencies include resilience and adaptability, which generally assumes self-awareness and the capacity to self-monitor, both of which are key to successful self-care and a meaningful medical career. However, they also assume a level of psychological maturity that for many people comes with age and life experience and that many prospective students do not have.

It is worth examining what specific advice on physician and student well-being is currently available to today's medical school applicants. The most comprehensive site of relevance is run by the AAMC, which features a number of interesting stories written by current medical students that advise applicants on multiple issues and describe the authors' own experiences. A good one to start with was posted by Jocelyn Carnicle, a second-year medical student at Texas Tech University Health Sciences Center El Paso, in September 2018, which says in part:

> Congratulations! Welcome to an exciting time and the beginning of a life-altering experience....It will be challenging though. You will spend so much time pouring over lectures that you may even start to dream about diagnoses as you attempt to get a peaceful night's sleep. Some days you will cry, and that is [okay]. The sheer volume of knowledge you must gain to be responsible for people's lives is terrifying. Find your support system and lean on them. You need to become comfortable with not knowing everything. This is harder than it sounds....Medical school is a marathon, not a sprint. You must be kind to yourself. Take study breaks to work out or cook a healthy meal. Learn to accept that not every single day will be a great study day, and even more importantly, learn when to call it quits. You need to have a life outside of studying....Lastly, I have to warn you, that some things will challenge you more than the heavy science load. You may question yourself and whether you belong at times. One of the hardest obstacles you will have to overcome in medical school and residency is the one inside your head. This is where I really need you to listen. My future colleague, you are not a fraud. You are a unique and capable individual with your own flaws just like me, just like everyone in your class, and you deserve to be here. (Carnicle 2018)

Reading Jocelyn's sensitive and insightful post, two issues stand out. The first is her passion and commitment, which are combined with a humble, thoughtful perspective whereby she recognizes the need to be socially broad and not excessively focused on work. Her post is a lesson for many medical school faculty and would have been a great document for Luis to read out, had he known of its existence. The second issue is her acceptance of the likelihood of psychological distress when she talks about the obstacles "inside your head" and the importance of maintaining a strong sense of purpose, something that is often lost in physicians who experience symptoms of burnout. Medical students in their first 2 years often describe the experience as being similar to trying to drink from a fire hose. Too much information must be learned, and most of it is not retained. This is a lesson that all physicians have to learn and understand, because it is physically impossible for anyone to keep up to date with the medical literature relevant to their areas of interest; too much is available. Those who wish to remain even close to current must adopt a habit of lifelong, "just in time" learning.

Interestingly, about half of all medical students make up their minds to go to medical school by the time they have left high school, just like Luis, and about half of those were confident of their future 5 years earlier. This Millennial generation of future doctors who have never experienced life without the internet has very different attitudes toward self-care and work-life balance than prior generations of physicians, and they are used to living a combination of in-person and online lives. Those who wish to attend medical school are increasingly aware that they need to keep their online profiles as clean and professional as possible, as Luis noted. This is something many partygoers find difficult; the ease of public posting on sites such as Facebook and Snapchat makes evidence of dubious or possibly misinterpreted behavior much more overt and easily available than in the past.

Not all admissions committees study applicants' social media accounts, but some certainly do, and every student should assume that he or she will be looked up online. The AAMC has a detailed review of how social media can affect a student's application to medical school (Association of American Medical Colleges 2019a) in which Luis E. Seija, a student member of the admission committee at Texas A&M College of Medicine, is quoted as saying,

> Applying to professional schools serves as, well, a lesson in professionalism and the development of a professional identity. Applicants should be aware that the latter often converges with the personal on social media. Admissions committees are not in the business of actively policing online personas or necessarily want to. However, it's not an uncommon practice to follow-up on information stated on a candidate's application (awards, blogs, etc.) with a simple internet search. (Association of American Medical Colleges 2019a)

This AAMC review is helpful, noting that a presence on some social media sites, such as LinkedIn, can be very positive. They recommend all students (and, of course, medical students and physicians) perform regular internet searches and contact sites to ask that they remove any posts or other information that may be prejudicial. Scott Rodgers, M.D., associate dean for student affairs at Vanderbilt University School of Medicine, sums up the dilemma best: "If students have any doubt about posting something on Facebook or any other social media site, then he or she should simply not do it. It is always best to err on the side of less rather than more" (Association of American Medical Colleges 2019a).

Moving on, what programs and behaviors may help students survive medical school and reduce the amount of burnout found within 2 years of entry? Research in this area is increasing, and the AAMC has developed an excellent set of tips for surviving medical school that Luis should surely read. These include (Association of American Medical Colleges 2019b)

1. Attend all the orientation programming
2. Identify and build relationships with mentors
3. Take an active role in your learning experience
4. Foster a team environment
5. Take care of your physical and mental health
6. Make time to explore career options
7. Realize the significance of joining the medical profession

All of these issues are important and are perhaps best summed up by ensuring that the medical school focuses on a healthy learning environment that includes good communication, supportive teams and groups—often involving the longitudinal colleges such as Luis described—and an emphasis on mentoring and self-care, as well as easy access to counseling and mental health care. Ideally, this climate will also include the use of pass/fail exams, as is currently being considered by the U.S. Medical Licensing Exam (USMLE), rather than the competitive scores that are required in the Step exams, as a way of reducing pressure on students. Strong financial support for students to reduce the worry of a heavy financial debt at graduation is also required, as I discuss in detail in Chapter 9. An example of a well-considered and detailed medical student wellness website replete with useful resources is that published by University of California, Davis (www.ucdmc.ucdavis.edu/mdprogram/student_wellness/index.html; University of California, Davis Health 2019). Had Luis reviewed this website, he would have found a wide range of resources as well as links to immediate support services, wellness events, childcare services, a monthly newsletter, and even monthly recipes.

Finally, moving on to Luis's vulnerability from a psychiatric perspective, and the implications of this vulnerability for his future career as a physician, one might ask why his ACE score is significant and what it means. In brief, the original ACE study measured 10 types of childhood trauma. Five were related to family members: a parent with alcoholism, a mother who is a domestic violence victim, a family member in jail, a family member diagnosed with a mental illness, and the disappearance of a parent through death, divorce, or abandonment. Five were personal: physical abuse, verbal abuse, sexual abuse, physical neglect, and emotional neglect. ACEs fall into three domains, namely, abuse (physical, emotional, and sexual), neglect (emotional and physical), and household dysfunction (substance abuse, divorce, violence, incarceration, and mental illness). The implications of this research, first published in 1998 after a large study by Kaiser in California (Felitti et al. 1998) and followed up by numerous other studies since, are substantial.

The many ACE studies are summarized at www.acestoohigh.com. In brief, they have shown that

- Childhood trauma is very common across all socioeconomic groups.
- A direct link exists between childhood trauma and the adult onset of chronic physical disease as well as depression, suicide, being violent, and being a victim of violence.
- The more types of trauma experienced in childhood, the higher the risk of health, social, and emotional problems.
- Most people usually experience more than one type of trauma—rarely is it only sexual abuse or verbal abuse—so childhood trauma can be seen as a vulnerability marker for later dysfunction.
- Exposure to early traumatic stress likely leads to abnormal brain development that affects sociocognitive skills and can lead to poor life decisions and choices in health habits.

Given this strong evidence of the link between childhood trauma and the adult onset of psychiatric disorders in particular, it is strange that so few studies have been done of ACEs in medical students and none has yet been published of ACEs in qualified physicians. An interesting study published in 2012 (Candib et al. 2012) that reviewed a number of early papers on the prevalence of abuse in physicians found that up to 42% of female physicians and 24% of male physicians had some experience of lifetime personal abuse, including witnessing violence between their parents. Unfortunately, this study did not measure ACEs. Some literature on ACEs in medical students and veterinary students is available; Sciolla et al. (2019), in a small study of 86 medical students, found that 44 reported at least one ACE and that 10, all female, reported exposure to four or more ACEs. This rate was similar to that in other populations studied, although the female bias was unusual. Strand et al. (2017) found that veterinary students reported being exposed to ACEs before age 18 at a rate similar to that of other population-based studies and concluded that these students did not enter the veterinary medical education system more at risk for poor mental health due to ACEs than the general population. In association with the Sacramento Sierra Valley Medical Society, Yellowlees et al. (submitted) have completed an as-yet unpublished study of 300 regional physicians whose ACE scores were slightly lower than community control subjects, but whose ACE scores did have a correlation with burnout levels, suggesting an association between ACESs and later burnout.

Why is the potential biological and psychosocial vulnerability of physicians so important, and why should the use of markers such as ACE scores be investigated to determine which future students and doctors may need more help and support? As is widely known, medical schools are working hard to diversify their classes and, in particular, to increase the admission of students from underserved communities, with the hope that the social and ethnic structure of future cohorts of physicians will more closely match those of the general population they are treating. While this overall objective is laudable, the potential unintended consequence is that this diversification may lead to increased numbers of future doctors who come from economically impoverished backgrounds that are associated with higher ACE scores than other populations. Such students would be more medically and psychiatrically vulnerable to burnout and other illnesses during their professional lives, as was the case for Luis. So although few would question the major potential benefits of changing the demography of doctors, some ethical questions arise from the possible introduction of more vulnerable individuals into the profession. These potentially vulnerable physicians will likely need extra help, support, and counseling to reduce their vulnerability from the start of their medical career and onward. This already happens for those students and future doctors who are physically disabled, such as blind or deaf, but who successfully live and practice as they overcome their disabilities and work effectively, so there is no reason why the same approach could not be taken for individuals with high ACE scores, especially if they come from economically impoverished environments.

We clearly need more research in this area, in both medical students and physicians, and we need to examine the ethics of what we do when we find that prospective physicians may be at increased risk of depression and substance use disorder, as well as suicide. Should we take action to try to prevent this, or to avoid it completely, perhaps even counseling very-high-risk trauma-exposed candidates not to apply to medical school? What is it that ultimately makes a good physician who thrives? What types of individuals should be targets for admissions committees and medical schools? Can we predict medical student or physician success at a lifestyle level? How do differing generations vary? We know that digital natives, who have never known life without the internet, have different learning styles and are more visual and "how-to" focused. What is the impact of early shadowing experiences, including scribing, and of all the sacrifices and delayed gratifications throughout a medical career, as discussed by Yellowlees (2018)? How should we adapt the medical school admissions process and in particular look for individuals who have already successfully "traveled a distance," to use a phrase borrowed from Dr. Kirch, the recent chair of AAMC? Finally, how do we pick students who will be able to work differently in the face of many future physician shortages and technological and policy changes? Do we need to recruit a different type of doctor for the future?

These are very difficult ethical and practical questions waiting for exploration and resolution.

References

Allegheny College: What are medical schools looking for? Health Professions (website). Meadville, PA, Allegheny College, 2019. Available at: https://sites.allegheny.edu/health/what-are-medical-schools-looking-for. Accessed April 10, 2019.

Association of American Medical Colleges: How Social Media Can Affect Your Application (website). Washington, DC, American Association of Medical Colleges, 2019a. Available at: https://students-residents.aamc.org/applying-medical-school/article/how-social-media-can-affect-your-application. Accessed April 10, 2019.

Association of American Medical Colleges: Tips for Surviving Medical School (website). Washington, DC, American Association of Medical Colleges, 2019b. Available at: https://students-residents.aamc.org/attending-medical-school/article/tips-surviving-medical-school. Accessed April 10, 2019.

Association of American Medical Colleges Staff: What medical schools are looking for: understanding the 15 core competencies. SDN: The Student Doctor Network, October 12, 2017. Available at: https://www.studentdoctor.net/

2017/10/12/what-medical-schools-are-looking-for-understanding-the-15-core-competencies. Accessed September 11, 2018.

Brazeau CM, Shanafelt T, Durning SJ, et al: Distress among matriculating medical students relative to the general population. Acad Med 89(11):1520–1525, 2014 25250752

Candib LM, Savageau JA, Weinreb L, et al: Inquiring into our past: when the doctor is a survivor of abuse. Fam Med 44(6):416–424, 2012 22733419

Carnicle J: Letter to an Incoming Medical Student (website). Washington, DC, American Association of Medical Colleges, 2018. Available at: http://aspiringdocsdiaries.org/a-letter-to-an-incoming-medical-student. Accessed September 10, 2018.

Dyrbye LN, West CP, Satele D, et al: Burnout among U.S. medical students, residents, and early career physicians relative to the general U.S. population. Acad Med 89(3):443–451, 2014 24448053

Eley DS, Leung J, Hong BA, et al: Identifying the dominant personality profiles in medical students: implications for their well-being and resilience. PLoS One 11(8):e0160028, 2016 27494401

Felitti VJ, Anda RF, Nordenberg D, et al: Relationship of childhood abuse and household dysfunction to many of the leading causes of death in adults. The Adverse Childhood Experiences (ACE) Study. Am J Prev Med 14(4):245–258, 1998 9635069

Gilbert LK, Breiding MJ, Merrick MT, et al: Childhood adversity and adult chronic disease: an update from ten states and the District of Columbia, 2010. Am J Prev Med 48(3):345–349, 2015 25300735

Hall D: Five med school application tips by the dean for admissions. Day in the Life, David Geffen School of Medicine, March 21, 2017. Available at: https://medschool.ucla.edu/body.cfm?id=1158&action=detail&ref=971. Accessed September 11, 2018.

Morris S: 5 key characteristics of successful medical school applicants. US News and World Report, April 5, 2016. Available at: https://www.usnews.com/education/blogs/medical-school-admissions-doctor/articles/2016-04-05/5-key-characteristics-of-successful-medical-school-applicants. Accessed April 5, 2016.

Sciolla A, Wilkes M, Griffin E: Adverse childhood experiences in medical students: implications for wellness. Acad Psychiatry 2019 30850989 Epub ahead of print

Strand EB, Brandt J, Rogers K, et al: Adverse childhood experiences among veterinary medical students: a multi-site study. J Vet Med Educ 44(2):260–267, 2017 28346049

University of California, Davis Health: Student Wellness (website). Sacramento, CA, University of California, Davis School of Medicine, 2019. Available at: http://www.ucdmc.ucdavis.edu/mdprogram/student_wellness. Accessed April 11, 2019.

Yellowlees P: Physician Suicide: Cases and Commentaries. Washington, DC, American Psychiatric Association Publishing, 2018

Yellowlees P, Misquitta R, Coates L, et al: The correlation of ACE scores and burnout in a community sample of physicians. Submitted for publication.

Chapter 6

MEDICAL SCHOOL: IMPLICIT BIASES AND A WELL-BEING CURRICULUM

Scenario

Dr. Harrod picked up the file for the first student on the day's interview list. He looked at the other three files on his desk and hoped that at least one of the four students he was seeing that morning would turn out to be an excellent prospect for the psychiatry residency program. Given that he and his colleagues were interviewing more than 80 medical students for just nine residency slots, he knew the chances were against that, but when he had read the files in detail the evening before, he had had a good feeling about the first student.

Dr. Harrod took his role as a faculty interviewer seriously, and as an ambitious, midlevel academic at associate professor level, he saw it as an opportunity to really help influence the success of the residency program. He had dressed more smartly than normal today, wearing his favorite navy-blue suit and turquoise silk tie. After all, the interview process was a two-way street: the student had to want to come to this residency program and the program had to want the student. Both parties had to impress each other. He turned to review the application packet on his knee.

Justin Raley's packet was impressive. As a final-year medical student, he was on the dean's honors list at his midwestern medical school and had a glowing letter of recommendation from the associate dean for students. He seemed to have strong leadership potential, having been class president and codirector of one of the four internal colleges at his medical school. His documents described several outside sports interests, mainly baseball and soccer, and he had been an active member of the national medical student association. He seemed to enjoy travel and before medical school had taken a number of trips to Europe and Asia as well as a month-long primary-care elective in Mexico. His personal statement, which described his rationale for applying to a psychiatry residency training program, was the only part of the packet that was surprising and unexpected, given that all other aspects of his academic and personal background seemed exemplary. Dr. Harrod knew that this would have to be the core topic of the upcoming interview.

A knock resounded on his door. Dr. Harrod checked his watch, adjusted his tie one last time, and got up from his chair to open the door.

"Good morning. I assume you are Justin Raley." He shook hands with the tall, slim, African American man. "Please come in. I am Dr. Harrod."

"Thank you," Justin responded. "I really appreciate you making yourself available to interview me, Dr. Harrod." Dr. Harrod motioned to Justin to take a seat in the slightly worn leather chair under the window. He collected Justin's application packet, a notepad, and pen and took his place in the other chair while looking Justin up and down carefully. He noted the candidate seemed fit and healthy and had short, clipped hair and attentive eyes. Justin was clean shaven and semicasually dressed in a light brown jacket, cream shirt, burgundy tie, dark brown corduroy trousers, and brown Sperry topsiders. He sat in a relaxed fashion, leaning comfortably back in the chair, having set his soft leather briefcase beside him on the carpeted floor.

"Let me also thank you for coming here for interviews, Justin. I know you've traveled a long way, and I hope you find it interesting and worthwhile. Did you enjoy the pizza night last night with our residents?"

"Yes. It was very kind of the department to arrange that social. All eight of us interviewees found it really interesting. It was great that six of the current residents were able to come. They were very positive about the program, and it was good to be able to ask them all sorts of practical questions about what happens here. I think I learned a lot. It's always reassuring to meet people who might in the future be colleagues as residents, because they can be honest about how they're treated and how the program works."

"What did you learn from them?" Dr. Harrod asked. "And remember, this interview is a two-way street: Having read your application packet, I have a number of topics I wish to discuss, and I assume you have your own questions for me as well. Please ask anything you want."

"Thanks, Dr. Harrod. I fully understand and appreciate your openness. What impressed me most about the residents was how supported they felt by everyone involved in the training program. This program has a reputation of being high quality and of producing first-class clinical psychiatrists with a strong background in multiple therapies as well as in psychopharmacology. The core aim is not to attempt to produce psychiatric researchers or highly biological psychiatrists, and they certainly backed up that opinion. That's good from my perspective, because my primary aim for doing a psychiatric residency is to become a first-class clinical psychiatrist. I wonder, Dr. Harrod, is that your view of the program?"

"I think that's a fair description, and it's pleasing to hear that we have that reputation. I have close experience of only two other residency programs, and certainly I think we pay a great deal more attention to the needs and health of our residents than they did."

"From your perspective, as a faculty member involved in teaching the residents, what do you think the department does to support residents, especially those from diverse backgrounds like me?" Justin continued.

"Well, we have the traditional supervision and mentoring that all training programs have, but I think one difference here is that we have very strong support from a large number of faculty and private-practice psychiatrists who themselves come from quite diverse social and ethnic backgrounds. Many of them have been teaching and supervising our residents for years. This provides great consistency of support for the residents and also lets them spend time with senior colleagues who have not taken the academic route after training and whose primary skills are clinical rather than on education or research. But let me focus on some of your interests first, and we can come back to this topic later."

"Certainly, Dr. Harrod." Justin replied.

"I'm fascinated by your decision to do psychiatry, especially because this seems a recent change; your medical student letters suggest that many of your supervisors expected you to go into surgery. I found it a bit difficult to work out the reasons for this change from your personal statement, although they seem mainly to relate to your experiences as a medical student and how you were educated. I wonder if you could explain in more detail why you wish to become a psychiatrist?"

Dr. Harrod had decided to be very direct because Justin was academically very strong and had the makings of a superb leader and physician. He genuinely wanted to understand Justin's change of career direction. He hoped the decision made sense and was easily explicable, because if it was, he expected to be able to strongly support Justin's application and to push for him to be accepted into the program. He was worried, however, because quite a few medical students whom he had interviewed had not had good reasons for going into psychiatry beyond simply academic interest, and the training program always looked for more than that.

Justin knew that this question would be coming and was not worried by it. He had decided to be completely open about his reasons for choosing psychiatry, and that if they did not meet the wishes of the training program, then so be it; he would try elsewhere. After all, he had had at least five interviews already, such was the strength of his academic profile.

"I appreciate you asking that up front Dr. Harrod, because I am well aware that this career direction was not something I was planning even a year ago. I have several reasons for the change, all of which seem to have come together at the same time. Actually, 5 years ago, if you had spoken to me as a college student, I would've told you I was thinking of doing psychology. I did a lot of research into professional careers and decided that rather than obtain a Ph.D. in psychology, I would be better to study medicine; if I was still interested in mental health at the end of medical school, I would do a residency in psychiatry afterward. So I went to medical school already thinking of psychiatry. However, I became enamored with surgery in the first year and thereafter focused mainly on that, doing elective research with, and obtaining mentoring from, a number of surgeons. I loved my surgery rotation as a third-year student, but I was rather put off by some of the cultural aspects of the surgical profession. For instance, the way the surgery attendings I worked with didn't support each other, even if an unexpected death occurred in the operating room. I was amazed by how they denied the impact of such an event on themselves and their colleagues. They seemed to be trained to just ignore this trauma and move to the next patient. But I still loved the surgery itself. Anyway, psychiatry was my last third-year rotation, and I was allocated to the hospital consultation service run by a very experienced psychiatrist."

"Was that your only rotation?" asked Dr. Harrod.

"No, I also went to an acute inpatient unit for a month, but the month I had with Dr. Losara was the most influential. Let me tell you why. The first thing I saw was how all the other physicians in the hospital, even the most independent and arrogant surgeons, enormously respected Dr. Losara. They would call him sometimes to ask about their patients, and he would frequently drop into the medical and surgical wards and join their rounds. One of the other students told me that in his outpatient practice Dr. Losara treated mainly physicians from all over the city. What was most interesting was how he worked in the hospital seeing consultations from all the medical and surgical teams. He kept telling us as students that his job was not only to help the patients referred to him but also to help the referring physicians or clinical teams and to make sure that they were properly educated about the psychiatric issues of their patients. His most famous saying, repeated by generations of students, was 'Remember, behind every patient referred to you is a physician asking for your help.' I soon worked out that he was helping a great many physicians, and it struck me that psychiatrists were the doctors best equipped to do that. That was a real insight for me and made me think back to why I had originally gone into medicine. When I was thinking of changing my mind and going into psychiatry, I went to speak to Dr. Losara on several occasions, and he was very supportive of my decision. Interestingly, he told me not to make this sort of decision purely on an intellectual rationale but to do what felt right to me and to listen to my inner feelings, which he called my 'gut feelings.' I've thought a lot about what he said, as a psychiatrist whom previously I would have expected to take a more psychological perspective, and I realized he was right. What I am doing simply feels right to me."

"I understand completely what you're saying, but was there anything else behind your change—beyond Dr. Losara's teachings and your past plans? It still seems a sudden, major change in your career direction," said Dr. Harrod.

"Certainly. A lot of things happen to medical students that never make it into their academic packets. Some of the things that happened to me as a medical student made me 100% sure that psychiatry is the right career for me."

"I see that you were very active in your group of students and in several medical student committees. Was this change related to those activities?"

"Partly, but there were other issues. Let me tell you about the influence my committee roles had first. I've always been involved in leadership activities. In high school, I was on a principal's student advisory committee, and in college I was heavily involved in student politics, usually focused on fees, student rights, and supporting the many diverse groups of students whom we felt needed more of a voice, such as the LGBT community. In medical school I volunteered to be a student representative on the curriculum committee for my first 2 years. That was fascinating because we were making big changes to the overall curriculum to make it more relevant to students. From my third year on, I've been on what we call the 'student progress committee,' which reviews students who are getting behind in their course, failing, or showing unprofessional behavior."

"That's a good combination of experiences. You must have learned a lot about medical education. But I'm not sure why that would turn you toward psychiatry," said Dr. Harrod.

"Well, as you know, the devil is always in the details. I'll summarize what I learned from being on the curriculum committee. The major task of the committee was to modernize our course after a fairly critical review by AAMC[1] at our last accreditation survey. I had to spend 2 years sitting through meetings that were essentially a fight between various groups of faculty, all of whom insisted they could not take any of their own teaching time out of the curriculum. They had been told to add new topics and competencies relevant to modern medicine, such as informatics, multimedia skills, genomics, communication skills, reasoning and big data analysis, business and organizational systems, human diversity, leadership, self-care, and physician well-being, to name a few. Several of the faculty on the committee, particularly those from anatomy and physiology, seemed especially powerful and were always better prepared than the clinical faculty, especially when it came to rules and regulations, but to me they seemed hopelessly out of date in terms of what information today's medical students need to learn. At one meeting, we actually got down to whether it was more important for students to know all the names of the bones of the foot or to understand how to recognize if a colleague is suicidal, and the 'bones of the foot' group won. Certainly we need to know about both, but not one over the other. I was frustrated, and so were all the other students when we passed on our reports of the meetings. Some of the events I witnessed

---

[1]AAMC=Association of American Medical Colleges.

on this committee made me quite disillusioned with medical school. I thought the aim was to create a curriculum designed to help train us to be the best doctors possible now and in the future, not doctors from a past century."

"I can understand that, Justin. Knowledge of the anatomy of the foot is important to learn, but so are the things you just mentioned. How does this relate to psychiatry?" said Dr. Harrod.

"We students finally put forward a list of topics that we thought needed to be in the curriculum, and the activity of the two psychiatrists on the committee was impressive. Along with a colleague from public health and another from internal medicine, they were the leaders for change and modernization of the curriculum, and they worked closely with us, supporting our requests. For instance, I brought up LGBT health care in the committee; I had been interested in that in college, and we had a number of medical students who were openly gay, both male and female. However, the reaction to my suggestion was generally fairly negative, and most of the faculty, although prepared to tolerate such topics in the curriculum, clearly were not enthusiastic. Once again, the two psychiatrists were helpful and met separately with me and my three student colleagues on the committee to plan a joint strategy for introducing a course on LGBT health, which I'm glad to say is going to start next year. After 2 years on that committee, I found that the psychiatrists seemed most open to change and modernization of the curriculum, including taking a more student-focused approach. They seemed to be listening to our ideas more and were less interested in just protecting their academic 'patch' like the others. But the past 18 months on the student progress committee have been even more influential on me."

"Interesting," said Dr. Harrod. "What happened there?"

"Well, as you know, all medical schools have these committees, and their job primarily is to review those students who are failing, on academic probation, or at risk of being dismissed from school. They deal with some very difficult situations, and a lot of their work is highly confidential, to the extent that the student members sometimes have to leave and are not given access to all the information about their colleagues. Unfortunately, as a member of this committee, I learned that medical school could be difficult sometimes for students who were not Anglo-Saxon whites, even in this day and age. My being black made people uncomfortable occasionally. I'm pretty sensitive to being treated differently because I'm black, and I can see it happening to others in subtle and not-so-subtle ways. This type of prejudice can be demoralizing. Then I tried to help one of my best friends at medical school who was struggling, but I failed in the end. That experience helped me decide that psychiatry was right for me, rather than surgery, so that I can work on preventing the things that happened to her from happening to medical students in the future," said Justin.

"That sounds very serious, Justin. Can you tell me broadly what happened and how it intersected with your decision to go into psychiatry? Are you talking about suicide, by any chance?"

"Yes, tragically. Janelle died 6 months ago of an overdose in her final year of medical school. And what happened to her was so preventable," Justin said sadly. "I've learned through hard experience that we need to look after ourselves as students and doctors a lot better than we have in the past."

"I am so sorry. What happened?"

"Well, Janelle was in the year above me, but we were in the same school-based internal college. She was assigned as my student mentor when I started medical school, and she was incredibly helpful. She took me under her wing, making sure I knew the best way to sign up for classes and understood the whole orientation process. She introduced me to lots of other people in our college group and made sure I had a smooth transition into school. We got on really well, and despite our many differences, we soon became good friends, socializing in the same group and sharing similar political views. Both of us had been politically active previously."

"What were your differences, Justin?" said Dr. Harrod. He was fascinated by Justin's story and very sensitive to the issue of suicide in medical professionals; an anesthesiologist colleague at the university had died from suicide the previous year.

"We could hardly have been more different. Janelle was a gay Hispanic woman who was former military. Before medical school, she had been a medic in Iraq and had done two tours of duty. She was very bright, and after her service she went back to school as a mature student and eventually obtained entry to medical school. Our school was close to a major military base, and a lot of ex-service people lived locally and were strongly encouraged to obtain degrees from the university. Each year of medical school had at least two or three students who were former military. It's something everyone was proud of—until Janelle's fate, that is, and the impact that her death had."

"Interesting. Here, when we think of diversity, we tend to only think of racial and ethnic differences, but the military component of diversity is also important, and I imagine that had an impact on the culture of the whole school," Dr. Harrod commented.

"That's correct. We were all proud of our military students and still are. But I'm not sure we actually do enough to support them. They often bear a burden we don't always recognize. I've learned that it's not enough to preach that we want to have diverse groups of students. We need to find better ways to identify and help their special needs."

"It sounds like she had some of those needs?" Dr. Harrod prompted.

"Yes, that's right. But it took me a long time to understand what Janelle's needs were. In retrospect, she was able to keep them well hidden during the first 2 years of the course, when we had little patient contact, but from the third year onward, the interactions with patients were just too much and seem to have opened a can of worms within her."

"What do you mean by that?"

"I'll explain in a moment, but first let me tell you about the first year that I knew her. Remember that, as a mature student in her early 30s and as a single, Hispanic, and openly gay female, she really stood out in a class that was mostly white or Asian. The school had only five black and three brown students in total, but because at least 30% of our students were Asian, it considered itself racially quite diverse. Incidentally, the racial variety of your residents and faculty is one of the reasons I would like to come here for residency." Justin paused. "Anyway, Janelle had strong views about LGBT students and decided she wanted to form an LGBT chapter of the American Medical Students Association at our school and, as the LGBT handbook from AMSA suggests, to try to 'paint the school pink.' I had some experience helping with such endeavors previously, although I'm straight. So I worked with her to set up the chapter, obtain faculty support, create a website, and recruit potential members who had already come out or were simply interested and supportive, as I was. This was why I was involved in suggesting more LGBT-relevant materials to the curriculum committee. She had helped me when I came to medical school, so it was only natural for me to help her on this."

"Now I see the connection. Good for you. That must have been quite a challenging process."

"It was, but more for Janelle than for me. She put a huge effort into it, and as a result, some of her grades fell and she failed the USMLE[2] Boards at the end of her second year, although she passed them on her next attempt. Failing the Boards, though, meant that she went on academic probation for a while, was reviewed by the student progress com-

---

[2]USMLE=United States Medical Licensing Examination.

mittee, and felt under extra pressure. This all happened a year before I joined the committee, and I remember her telling me how threatening she found the whole process—not the least bit supportive, which was the theoretical aim of the committee. At the same time, she was clearly gaining a reputation for herself among the faculty, and not a good one, because she was typical ex-military—unsubtle and direct, challenging teachers and attendings if they didn't teach well. She wasn't threatened by authority, generally, but was very respectful of those who were not threatened by her and whom she felt deserved her respect. All this meant that by the time she went into her third-year classes she was, to a certain extent, marked. When it became clear that she was not very good with some patients and became unusually anxious with patients who had been through traumas, especially gunshots, motor vehicle accidents, rapes, and other violent incidents, she was in trouble. She failed her surgical and OBGYN[3] rotations outright, but luckily, her third rotation was psychiatry. She started with Dr. Losara, and within a few days he had taken her aside and met with her at length. She had broken down in tears while presenting a patient to him who had been a victim of incest, and she had then become very angry and walked off the ward."

"That sounds very difficult, indeed. I assume she had some sort of anxiety or PTSD,[4]" Dr. Harrod observed. "What happened next?"

"Well, I ended up seeing her later that evening, and she finally opened up to me, telling me things she said she was ashamed of and had never told anyone else. It was me who encouraged her to go back and speak to Dr. Losara, even though at that stage I only knew him by reputation as being a very caring physician."

"What sort of things had happened to her? It sounds as though you were being put in a difficult situation."

"The long and short of it is that she did have severe PTSD that she had tried desperately to hide and cover over. She told me she had had a few therapy sessions and been put on medication before she left the military. She thought she had her symptoms under control and could manage medical school, but when she came into contact with traumatized patients, her symptoms returned. She'd been involved in a whole series of dreadful incidents in Iraq, with friends being blown up and killed by IEDs,[5] but the trauma that most affected her was what she called 'MST,' or military sexual trauma. She never told me all the details,

---

[3]OBGYN=obstetrics and gynecology.
[4]PTSD=posttraumatic stress disorder.
[5]IEDs=improvised explosive devices.

but as a female, she was a target of a senior officer who had raped her on several occasions. The military apparently closed ranks when she finally complained, and it wasn't until she left the theater of war that she received treatment, although that was mainly focused on the IED-related traumas because she talked little about the sexual ones. She kept telling me how ashamed she was to be in this situation and how it felt as though it was her fault for having become a victim of MST, and how she must have done something wrong to deserve it." Justin sat back, slowly reflecting. "That was the first time I'd ever really heard anyone tell such a story. Remember, I was still in my second year at this stage and had had little contact with patients, so I really didn't know what to do beyond listen and be sympathetic and suggest she seek help from the student health services. I felt really lacking in the skills or knowledge of how to help her." Justin came to a halt and looked up at Dr. Harrod, who was listening sympathetically and attentively.

"What happened after that?" said Dr. Harrod.

"Well, Janelle did see a psychiatrist for a few sessions at the medical school. I found out that the school pays for two psychiatrists to spend a total of 3 days per week just seeing medical students, as well as for several psychologists to provide therapy. Don't you think it's bizarre that medical schools, who take the best and brightest students, have to provide that amount of mental health support for their students? It really shows that something is very wrong with the educational process and culture in medical schools. I don't know any law schools that have in-house psychiatrists." Justin stopped for a moment. "Sorry, I will try to keep to the topic, but it is weird, don't you think?"

"That's one way of looking at it," answered Dr. Harrod thoughtfully. "But most medical schools, including ours, automatically provide a lot of mental health support and treatment for their students. It seems to have just become expected and essential. We learned a long time ago how important it is to provide these services to students and staff."

Justin nodded. "Anyway, Janelle helped me make my decision to become a psychiatrist. She struggled through the rest of her third year but had to repeat her surgery and OBGYN rotations as directed by the student progress committee, which I joined about that time. I didn't hear the discussions about her in the committee, but she told me that she thought that the committee was a constant threat to her, and she was terrified of any meetings she had with them. She usually met just with the chairperson, but she knew how much power they had over her. She told me in confidence once that the committee reminded her of a military tribunal and that every time she had contact with them, her PTSD symptoms, especially her impaired sleep, became worse for several days. I know that she was supposed to continue seeing a psychiatrist during that year, but she didn't always keep the appointments. She said she stuck to the medications, but I don't think she continued with the therapy. She was afraid of being absent from her rotations. To have therapy she would have to be off the wards for 3 hours per week for a single session, and she thought that was too much. I know that some of this was her fault, but she thought she could manage things herself. Because she had failed two rotations, her usual group of supportive student friends had moved on, so she became more isolated while trying to repeat the rotations. In the last year of her life, I and the others involved in the LGBT chapter, which she chaired, became her main support system, sort of by default, and that proved to be yet another stressor for her."

"It sounds to me like that would have given her a really positive sense of purpose," suggested Dr. Harrod. "What changed?"

"In theory you're right, of course, and that's what I also thought right up to the end, when she died. In retrospect, however, I think it was actually a bad thing for her to do because of the implicit biases she kept encountering among both students and faculty. She needed more help than we could provide."

"That sounds very unfortunate, and I can see that this weighs heavy on you still," Dr. Harrod said.

"Yes, I feel bad that she didn't get the help she needed. The more energy and effort she put into developing the LGBT chapter, the more critical people became about her efforts and the more angry and distressed she became. Looking back, I think she somehow thought that if she could get the chapter up and running, and accepted by the medical school establishment, that somehow that magically would validate her existence and make people accept her more. Maybe she was putting all her energy into the chapter to deflect from dealing with her own internal struggles, which were really tearing her apart. I remember a few months before her death, sitting down with her one evening and trying to persuade her to stop focusing so much on LGBT issues and instead to spend more time on her clinical work to improve her grades on the rotations she was taking. We had a really long talk about it, and she just couldn't see how stopping or reducing her LGBT crusade—which it was by that stage—would be possible, because of the potential loss of pride it would entail. She had focused excessively on it, to the detriment of her work, which led to her failing another rotation and having more trouble with the committee on student progress."

Justin sat back, looking troubled. He was not sure if he should go on with his story, but he decided to persist because it was so important to him and to why he wanted to become a psychiatrist.

"This is where I think the medical school may have failed Janelle. I think they had gotten to the stage where they were simply fed up with her. She was failing her rotations and was at times quite disruptive, with her focus on LGBT issues to the exclusion of almost everything else, but it was also quite evident to me, and to many of other students, that she was not well. She constantly talked about her military experiences and became excessively angry with anyone in authority, especially males. Whenever she had to take an oral examination, if her examiner was a full professor, she became very anxious; her fear of powerful men, in particular, kept reminding her of her experience of MST. At times she was quite paranoid and refused to accept that any of her academic failures were her own fault, blaming everyone else instead—the nurses on the wards, the patients for not giving good histories, and particularly the attendings and faculty for being out to trick her. She became convinced that this was because she was Hispanic and gay, although in my view, the school community, if anything, overcompensated in its attempts not to discriminate against her in any way." Justin looked up to make sure Dr. Harrod was following. Satisfied, he went on.

"By the middle of her fourth year, it had become common knowledge that she was probably unwell. We students all assumed she had relapsed and had more symptoms of PTSD. Yet, at the same time, she was making racist accusations to a number of people and had become very unpopular with her teachers, some of whom felt that they were unable to teach her in an honest way for fear she would file a complaint against them on the basis of either gender or racial discrimination. At least, that's what I heard after her death, although I don't think she actually made any formal complaints. Whenever she was brought before the committee, she made discriminatory comments that caused a lot of disquiet. The sad part is that her behavior made people afraid of her. She was intimidating. She even shouted at me a couple of times, telling me not to interfere and that she would manage everything herself. I will never forget the two discussions we had about her on the committee, where it was obvious that the chair, a kindly pediatrician, was afraid of talking to her. In the end he did speak to her, with another faculty member from the committee present, but they both treated her with kid gloves, not wanting to upset her or suggest that she might be unwell. This went on for several months—Janelle distressed, angry, confrontative, and paranoid, and the school community withdrawing from her, intimidated, and afraid to confront her or take any action, just hoping she would somehow pass her exams and eventually move on from medical school."

"Surely someone must have taken her aside and tried to discuss her situation with her," Dr. Harrod commented. "It sounds to me like she needed to have some time off and proper psychiatric treatment. How come that didn't happen?"

"You know, I will really never know the answer to that question. Remember, I'm just a medical student, and I have no idea what the faculty may have done. It's my impression that they did very little. They should have seen that she was sick and forced her to take time off and get treatment. They would have done so if she'd had a broken leg, but they all avoided her because her problem was psychiatric. What sort of a profession, especially in a medical school, doesn't look after its own when they're sick? She wasn't fit to be seeing patients. She told me that she wasn't going back to her psychiatrist again and that her medications were of no use, even though I thought she had been better when taking them and told her so. She said therapy had helped her early on, before she came to medical school, but insisted that she wasn't able to attend therapy with her fourth-year class schedule and the need to travel to other hospitals and clinics. I did ask her if she thought taking some time off would be worthwhile, but she disagreed, saying she couldn't afford to because she already had much more student debt than she had originally expected to have. She just kept saying that she would soldier on with her course, and with organizing the LGBT chapter, and would get through eventually. I never even thought of her committing suicide, because despite everything, she still seemed so strong. I regret not asking her about that directly, as I know I should have."

"What eventually happened to her? How did she die?"

"It was both tragic and dramatic. A bit like she had lived—larger than life. She was on a month's emergency medicine rotation at a hospital 50 miles away from the school, so she was isolated from people like me who were still trying to keep in close contact with her. Only three of us from the original LGBT committee were left because she had driven the others away with her anger and blaming. After her suicide, an investigation found she had not been doing well on her rotation and had had several disputes over patient care with the emergency department physicians. It seems that she was doing the same with them as she had been doing on other rotations: projecting and blaming everyone else for the patient's problems and accusing staff of discrimination against her and several patients. But there was more, it turns out. When her case files were reviewed after her death, it seems that she had seen two recent rape cases, and in those cases her notes were very extensive and angry, very different from a professional note. The inquest concluded that she was likely depressed, suffering from PTSD and confusing her own experiences of MST with what had happened to these patients, which triggered more of her symptoms." Justin broke off from his chain of thought, reflecting on a difficult time. "The Saturday after her third week of the rotation, when she was not due to be working, she went to the local military cemetery. I didn't know that this cemetery existed, but apparently it was where several people from her military corps were buried. She went wearing her full-dress uniform and walked around the cemetery for an hour or so, chatting with some other veterans and their families, seemingly friendly and relaxed. At peace with herself. Then, late in the afternoon, she stood at attention in front of the grave of one of her friends, took her gun out of its holster, and calmly shot herself in the head. She was seen by other visitors, who rushed over to her, but it was too late. In her jacket pocket were two letters—one to her mother, in which, among other things, she apologized for not having been a better daughter, and one to the three of us who were still part of her LGBT chapter and had stuck with her throughout medical school."

"My goodness. That is tragic," said Dr. Harrod.

"Yes, it was," said Justin. "And after the inquest and an internal investigation, the school acknowledged that it could have done more to help her. From what I understand, they are currently planning on including more training about self-care and the recognition of psychiatric problems for both faculty and students. But it was the letter that Janelle wrote that had the biggest impact on me. She knew that I was thinking of doing psychiatry and that I had not liked the culture I found in surgery. She said in her letter, very simply, that if I had been a psychiatrist, she would have been happy to come see me. She wrote that she thought I was caring and concerned for my colleagues and that she had always been impressed by how I had aligned myself with her LGBT friends, even though I was not personally gay, because that showed how sympathetic I was to groups that were frequently marginalized and victimized. She admitted that she knew she would be dealing with her mental illness forever and that this extra stigma, on top of being discriminated against for being brown and gay, was too much for her. The stigma of psychiatric disorder in someone who wanted to be a physician was too much; she couldn't see continuing her life like that, so she felt her only option was to end it."

Commentary

This chapter is really about Janelle, an increasingly unwell medical student who eventually died from suicide, as seen through the lens of her younger colleague, Justin, as he is applying for residency. Both Janelle and Justin were likely on the receiving end of a raft of discrimination and implicit biases at medical school, eventually leading Justin to choose a residency program where these were less likely to occur. The other concepts of importance in the chapter are the need for diversity—racial, ethnic, and attitudinal—among medical students and faculty and how to provide care and support for some of these diverse groups, as well as the importance of including such topics in the medical school curriculum. Finally, the scenario demonstrates a need for some doctors to become expert in treating other doctors and medical students, as Dr. Losara did. Incoming medical students have less burnout and depression and higher level of resilience than age-matched peers, as discussed in Chapter 2, yet we know from the literature that by the second year of medical school, medical students are doing worse on burnout indices than their peers, that nearly 30% of medical students endorse symptoms of depression, and that one in nine have suicidal ideation (Yellowlees 2018). We also know that distress in medical students is associated with less professional behavior and less empathy, so they clearly need to receive help, and psychiatrists seem to be an ideal group who are clinically well trained to take on this task (see Chapter 7).

So what do we know about culture, discrimination, implicit biases, and awareness about these important cultural issues in both medical students and their teaching faculty? And how has the selection process for medical schools changed over the past decade as a starting point to providing a solution for some of these difficult issues? How can we improve the processes currently in place to enable students to seek care for themselves and to make good career choices? As physicians, we like to think that we are always fair and egalitarian in our interactions with our patients and our colleagues. Unfortunately, this is simply not true.

What, then, is implicit bias? Why is it so important in health care? And why did this likely lead to some of the difficulties experienced by Janelle and Justin? In brief, *implicit biases* are unconscious associations we all make that lead us to negatively evaluate someone else based on characteristics such as race or gender. FitzGerald and Hurst (2017) explored this issue in detail in a fascinating systematic review of the literature. They found that health professionals at all stages of their careers exhibit the same levels of implicit bias as the wider population—despite the core professional and ethical assumption that all patients, no matter what their background, should receive the same level of treatment and care. They found that the sociodemographic characteristics of physicians and nurses were correlated with the level of bias and that this affected treatment decisions of all types. The most common biases found related to gender, color, ethnicity, nationality, and sexual orientation, but studies involving health care professionals have also found biases against people with Middle Eastern– or African American–sounding names, the mentally ill, people who are overweight, and those who are economically poor. FitzGerald and Hurst concluded that the health care profession needs to address the role of implicit biases in disparities in health care and to reduce the inherent prejudices and the tendency to stereotype both patients and colleagues such as Janelle experienced, to her detriment.

Given this background, it is not surprising that Janelle and Justin had a hard time setting up an LGBT chapter at medical school, although some very helpful resources are available that they could have consulted. The organization Health Professionals Advancing LGBTQ Equality (previously known as the Gay and Lesbian Medical Association) has an excellent website (glma.org). The American Medical Students Association's (2019) Committee on Gender and Sexuality, for instance, has produced a well-thought-out guide on how to "Paint Your School Pink" for student leaders who want to start an LGBT medical student organization at their school, as was mentioned in the scenario. This guide provides essential instruction and advice for student leaders as well as links to projects and resources on topics ranging from promoting institutional and curriculum change to mentorship and strengthening student organizations. Information is available for students who wish to work in this area and create local chapters, including a very useful series of 10 recommended steps to take to set up a local chapter (American Medical Students Association 2019):

1. Find an administrative or faculty advisor
2. Assemble founding members
3. Start a confidential mailing list
4. Name the group
5. Determine the group's mission
6. Affiliate your group with your school's AMSA chapter
7. Seek advice on the LGBT climate at your school; notify administration about your group, but do not ask permission to create it
8. Find funding through events and administration

9. Keep records of your group's leaders and activities
10. Have fun and do great advocacy work

Unfortunately, Janelle's illness, and her aggressive approach, likely contributed to the failure of the LGBT chapter. It would have been much easier for her if she had had a mentor who could support her more thoroughly and, in particular, have taught her more about the impact of implicit bias (and, of course, sometimes explicit bias) and how this can counteract change in groups and systems.

This concept of implicit bias and solutions for its consequences are starting to attract some interesting research. Hall et al. (2015) described how such bias influences health care outcomes adversely. In their review, they concluded that most health care providers appear to have implicit biases on the basis of color, with positive attitudes toward whites and negative toward blacks. These researchers focused on some possible solutions, noting that health care providers in some disciplines, such as pediatrics, tended to exhibit less implicit bias. They suggested that reexamination of the curricula and comparisons by specialty might be useful and that interventions for bias may have to be different according to the needs of particular specialties.

Solutions to the problem of implicit bias are sorely needed, and this issue has been addressed by the Institute for Healthcare Improvement (IHI; IHI Multimedia Team 2017) and The Joint Commission (2016). The IHI has developed a list of strategies that can be used to reduce implicit bias and should be included in all medical school and residency programs. These include the following (IHI Multimedia Team 2017):

- Perspective taking—put yourself in the other person's shoes
- Individuation—see the other person as an individual rather than as a stereotype
- Stereotype replacement or opposite imaging—recognize a stereotypical response and imagine the individual as the opposite of this stereotype
- Increase your contact with people from stereotyped groups, especially socially
- Partnership building—reframe the interaction as an equal collaboration

Others seeking solutions have emphasized the importance of understanding different cultures and social groupings as well as recognizing the power of unconscious bias and situations that may magnify stereotyping behavior. All of these topics should be included as core learning material in any medical school curriculum and as part of any professionalism training program for physicians and other health care providers at all stages of their careers.

Caroline Elton (2018), in her sensitive and insightful book on the inner lives of doctors, made the point that only the psychological needs of one half of the doctor–patient dyad have been widely recognized—those of the patient. She described how doctors' psychological needs are denied, ignored, or not even considered, suggesting that a systemic "psycholectomy" has been performed on the profession as a whole. In my previous book (Yellowlees 2018), I explored and examined the psychodynamic upbringing of many physicians, noting their tendency to develop delayed gratification as a habit and lifestyle, with many physicians preferring to sacrifice present-day rewards for future potential gains. Of course, this means that doctors inevitably become used to living less in the moment and learn to ignore their unconscious needs, leading to a tendency to be more subject to the implicit biases held by all of us.

It is important to focus on teaching about implicit bias in medical school and residency and to educate physicians about bringing these biases to a conscious level, but what about the impact of implicit bias on faculty who have never been so trained, particularly with regard to the medical school admissions process? We know historically, as Elton (2018) described, that approximately half of U.S. medical students come from the top 20% income bracket, whereas only 5% are from the bottom 20% bracket, so these social backgrounds are emblematic of today's faculty. Most medical schools are changing in alignment with AAMC admissions initiatives and are attempting to increase the diversity of their classes so the population of future doctors will eventually more closely parallel the national population from a gender, ethnic, and racial perspective. Given the current faculty population, however, this can hardly be done using traditional interview methods where white faculty have tended to choose white students.

Two major approaches to this, ideally performed together, are 1) training faculty in implicit bias so that they change their selection behaviors, and 2) changing the traditional admissions process to medical school.

Capers (2019) described the process of implicit bias training for faculty at Ohio State University College of Medicine. When it was introduced in 2012, all members of the admissions committee were required to take various implicit associations tests. The results showed that many committee members exhibited implicit white race preference, implicit bias against homosexuals, and unconscious associations of men with "career" and women with "homemaker." This led to the development of annual implicit bias mitigation workshops and to the admission of a significantly more diverse medical student population. Capers described how the following educational interventions have since become routine:

1. The admissions dean leads two half-hour implicit bias workshops each year for the entire medical center community.
2. Annual, mandatory implicit bias mitigation training sessions are provided for all application screeners and admissions committee members, who participate in 45-minute moderated discussions of implicit bias vignettes and evidenced-based strategies to reduce bias.
3. Recommended research readings on implicit bias are provided to the admissions committee and included in the admissions committee manual.
4. An interview-day "cheat sheet" that reviews a bulleted list of strategies to reduce implicit bias is provided to all interviewers.

The second major approach to reducing the impact of implicit bias is to change the medical school admissions process so that it is not so dependent on the results of one or two interviews between students and faculty, as has been the case historically. Eva et al. (2004, 2018) at McMaster University in Canada have developed a multiple mini-interview (MMI) format that has now been adopted by most U.S. medical schools and many other schools worldwide. This format consists of 10 stations lasting 8 minutes each, with 2-minute intervals between them where evaluators can complete standardized evaluation forms and candidates can read about the next station. Each candidate is therefore observed for about 80 minutes by eight evaluators performing a wide range of tasks, both individual and team based, including problem solving and interviewing, communications skills, and decision making. As an MMI evaluator, I have observed students—opposite trained actors playing various roles—help a person with alcoholism reduce his smoking and alcohol consumption, help an anxious work colleague with a flying phobia get on a plane, and apologize to an angry motorist whose car they have just dented. These are excellent tests of decision making and empathy. I have seen other students solve problems that involve teamwork, creativity, leadership, and collaboration before they are tested on ethical responses to situations or prove their capacity for critical thinking by rapidly reviewing some marketing materials. Unfortunately, I have also seen candidates being insensitive, callous, uncaring, and dismissive, all traits we do not wish to see in future doctors and that may be hard to detect in the traditional one-on-one interview. The MMI interview processes are much more objective than traditional interviews and seem to markedly reduce the opportunity for the implicit biases of faculty to affect the outcomes, so they are increasingly becoming standard practice. This is good, but the question remains: Why is the MMI not being used in other areas of medicine, such as at entry to residency, where traditional one-on-one interviews are still primarily used?

Moving back to the scenario, how best can mental health care, as well as counseling regarding career choices and decisions, be provided for medical students? How can the topic of self-care and the care of colleagues become core to the curricula of medical schools? All medical schools have administrative faculty whose role it is to provide such career, support, and decision-making services, and most provide medical students with access to counselors, psychologists, and psychiatrists for mental health assessment and treatment. A number of schools, such as the University of California (UC) Davis, also provide students with access to online tools that allow them to self-assess for depression, anxiety, substance abuse, and suicidality (Yellowlees 2018) and with useful online resource pages (University of California, Davis Health 2019). The UC Davis website is a good example of a comprehensive program of support and triaging for medical students, with regular blogs on wellness and sections and links on counseling and support services, crisis intervention, wellness events, stories, and resources as well as some with a focus on military careers and military mentors, as well as regular newsletters.

The AAMC, whose members comprise all 147 accredited U.S. and 17 accredited Canadian medical schools, is taking a lead in this area and has issued a statement on clinician well-being that summarizes their perspective as follows:

> The AAMC is committed to enhancing patient care and welfare, and to the belief that the optimal delivery of care requires an environment where all health care providers can thrive; where faculty, staff, and learners feel supported and well treated; where diversity, inclusion, and health equity are promoted; and where patients are empowered to make informed health care decisions. (Association of American Medical Colleges 2019)

Although as yet no formal, national "well-being curriculum" has been developed that can be widely implemented in medical schools, I have described the beginning of a framework for such a curriculum (Yellowlees 2018) and mentioned several topics discussed in the scenario here. The following topics comprise an extended version of this original framework and should be considered for inclusion in all medical school curricula:

- Regular participation in process-oriented reflective small groups and membership of multiyear internal colleges that provide student peer-support and mentoring
- A wide range of mentoring and mentee supervision opportunities so that these become part of the post–medical school culture (see Chapters 3 and 4)
- Ways of creating opportunities to strengthen professional and social relationships and to network widely and appropriately
- Career planning and creation of individual development plans (see Chapter 4)
- Decision making and clinical reasoning that takes into account future changes in medicine, such as the need for physicians to be expert in large data analysis and pattern matching as well as excellent diagnosticians who can take into account massively increasing and disparate datasets (see Chapter 8)
- Content on the various specific psychiatric, substance abuse, and personality disorders that affect physicians and how to recognize and treat them in any physician, including the individuals themselves
- Content and discussion of personal identity development and transformation, the interaction between burnout and physician health (including suicidal thoughts and behaviors), empathy, compassion, resiliency, and how to become reflective practitioners
- Active participation and learning about resilience, mindfulness, exercise, nutrition, communication. and relationships
- Instruction about organizational systems and the interactions that occur within them, and an understanding of institutional awareness and resources that can be used to change institutions
- Specific skills development in interpersonal professional relationships
- Modules and discussion groups on caring and compassionate leadership, financial, and business skills
- Media training, combined with experiential training using multiple communications technologies with patients and colleagues

Many of these topics are being introduced at individual medical schools, perhaps even in place of anatomy at some, but a comprehensive curriculum in well-being is still lacking anywhere. For how long will this continue?

References

American Medical Students Association: Paint your school pink, in LGBT Handbook. Chantilly, VA, American Medical Students Association, 2019. Available at: https://www.amsa.org/advocacy/action-committees/gender-sexuality/lgbt-handbook. Accessed May 2, 2019.

Association of American Medical Colleges: AAMC Statement on Commitment to Clinician Well-Being and Resilience. Washington, DC, Association of American Medical Colleges, 2019. Available at: https://www.aamc.org/download/482732/data/aamc-statement-on-commitment-to-clinician-well-beingandresilience.pdf. Accessed May 2, 2019.

Capers QIV: Rooting out implicit bias in admissions. AAMC News, February 5, 2019. Available at: https://news.aamc.org/diversity/article/rooting-out-implicit-bias-admissions. Accessed May 5, 2019.

Elton C: Also Human: The Inner Lives of Doctors. New York, Basic Books, 2018

Eva KW, Rosenfeld J, Reiter HI, et al: An admissions OSCE: the multiple mini-interview. Med Educ 38(3):314–326, 2004 14996341

Eva KW, Macala C, Fleming B: Twelve tips for constructing a multiple mini-interview. Med Teach 41(5):510–516, 2018 29373943

FitzGerald C, Hurst S: Implicit bias in healthcare professionals: a systematic review. BMC Med Ethics 18(1):19, 2017 28249596

Hall WJ, Chapman MV, Lee KM, et al: Implicit racial/ethnic bias among health care professionals and its influence on health care outcomes: a systematic review. Am J Public Health 105(12):e60–e76, 2015 26469668

IHI Multimedia Team: How to reduce implicit bias. IHI Improvement Blog, September 28, 2017. Available at: http://www.ihi.org/communities/blogs/how-to-reduce-implicit-bias. Accessed April 29, 2019.

The Joint Commission: Implicit bias in health care. Quick Safety (23), April 2016. Available at: https://www.jointcommission.org/assets/1/23/Quick_Safety_Issue_23_Apr_2016.pdf. Accessed April 29, 2019.

University of California, Davis Health: Student Wellness (website). Sacramento, CA, University of California, Davis School of Medicine, 2019. Available at: http://www.ucdmc.ucdavis.edu/mdprogram/student_wellness. Accessed May 3, 2019.

Yellowlees P: Physician Suicide: Cases and Commentaries. Washington, DC, American Psychiatric Association Publishing, 2018

Website of Interest

Health Professionals Advancing LGBTQ Equality website: www.glma.org

Chapter 7

RESIDENCY: A NARCOTIC ADDICT'S NEW CAREER

Scenario

I walked into the waiting room to find my new patient. I knew what he looked like, having scanned the emergency department (ED) residency list and seen Dr. Asim Chofan's image and biography beforehand. In the photo, my new patient was a rather young-looking Asian man with buzz-cut black hair. He was clean shaven, with a round face, and seemed somewhat overweight. In the photo he had worn a white shirt, a lavender tie, and a white lab coat that proudly showed his name. I was looking forward to meeting Dr. Chofan after my fascinating discussion with his training director. She had finished our conversation by saying that when he had started residency, he was the last person she would have expected to be referring for psychiatric assistance, but she now couldn't see him succeeding without substantial help, whatever was wrong with him.

I looked around the busy waiting room, where more than a dozen patients were waiting to be seen. I saw no one who looked similar to the photo, presumably taken 3 years ago when he started residency. The only young Asian male in the room was standing nervously by the front door, almost as though he were ready to escape. He was thin, with greasy black hair, and dressed in worn-out jeans, a faded tee shirt, and a black leather jacket despite the heat of the day. I had to take a second look before I realized it was Asim. I called his name to be sure it was him, and when he replied in the affirmative, I asked him to follow me to my clinic room.

My room, like those used by many psychiatrists in major medical centers, is very conventional. In and out boxes had papers sticking out here and there. Three computer screens, which I use for all of my writing and editing as well as for seeing patients via telemedicine, are equally spaced across the back of the large desk. About half of my patients prefer to be seen at home or their workplace by video to avoid traveling to my clinic, especially my physician patients. I invited Asim to sit in one of my leather chairs while I took the other. I noticed him taking his time to check the various picture frames around the room that held a combination of degree documents, prints, and paintings collected over many years of practice.

I began the session. "Thanks for coming to see me, Dr. Chofan. I understand that your training director, Dr. Brucer, has talked to you about coming to see me and is very concerned about you." To this Asim slumped into his chair, looking downward toward his feet and saying nothing. Finally, he nodded his head.

"I don't know why she insists I see you. Everyone knows that I have chronic pain in my back from ankylosing spondylitis and that I need to take pain medication. I just took one tablet too many the other night by mistake, and that's why I seemed a bit off at work. I have no reason to see you. You just need to talk to my primary care doc to have him confirm my situation. I have no idea why I'm seeing a psychiatrist."

"Well, given that you're uncertain why you're here, perhaps I should tell you what Dr. Brucer has told me. Incidentally, I've already looked at your medical record and have seen all the notes and X rays confirming your back problems. It does seem clear that you have longstanding chronic pain, which is rotten. I am so sorry," I said.

"Exactly," he responded. "That's why this is a waste of time. But yes, please tell me what Dr. Brucer said. I'm very interested to hear what her accusations are. She's not interested in my health, just in making sure that we residents cover all our shifts and that patients get seen quickly."

"I'll summarize our discussion," I told him. "She told me that you've missed three shifts altogether in the past month and been late on four other occasions, and you haven't been able to give a good explanation for any of these events. This is apparently on top of longstanding tardiness and your deteriorating academic performance on the internal residency quizzes, which she said has led to you receiving two letters of expectation in the past year. Dr. Brucer also told me that she and other attendings have been observing you carefully at work and are concerned that you might be taking too many painkillers for your back pain, concluding on several occasions that you seemed to be either excessively sedated or possibly somewhat high. On top of this, she told me you've lost a lot of weight in the past year, about 30 pounds by her estimate, and she wondered if you were not eating properly. I'm sure you can understand her concerns about your health. She decided that I should see you before you go back to work as planned next week."

"All of that is explained, as I said, by my back pain," replied Dr. Chofan, rather irritably. "Why do none of you listen?"

"Let's start with your back pain, then," I answered. "Tell me about it, and what you do to cope."

"What I do depends on where I am. If I'm at work, I take very little Oxycontin and try to just grin and bear the pain. But I find that difficult, so in the past few months I've been trying to take the Oxycontin regularly, every 2 hours, whether I'm working or not."

"That means you must be taking a minimum of 12 tablets every day, by your counting," I said. I had logged into the state's controlled-substances database earlier that morning to review all the prescriptions Asim had picked up in the past year, so I knew he was taking a lot more Oxycontin than he was telling me. He had prescriptions not only from his own primary care physician but also from three other doctors at urgent care centers whom he seemed to visit fairly regularly.

I continued the discussion. "Are you sure that's all you've been taking, Dr. Chofan? The story from Dr. Brucer suggests more, and when I checked the state controlled-substances database, what I found indicates you're getting several times that amount from four separate doctors. Can you explain that?" Asim just looked down. No response. No eye contact. Only his right leg shaking and trembling suggested any impact of my words. I waited for a short while before deciding to continue. "It seems to me that you may have a much more serious drug problem than you've been admitting and are likely addicted to narcotics. Do you think that might explain your behavior recently? Would you like to tell me more about what's been going on?"

The consultation continued in this vein. It was like pulling teeth; he remained very defensive and elusive, difficult to tie down to hard facts. The story, as he told it to me initially, was approximately as follows.

Asim Chofan came from a high-achieving Asian family where educational success was key. His father was also a doctor, a successful surgeon, and his mother ran a public relations company and was quite a high-profile member of the local community, involved with numerous charities and community development projects and often in the media. He was the second of two sons; his elder brother was a corporate lawyer on a fast track to senior management. Asim had always loved arts and music, with real talent as a painter and a love of playing the violin, but his father in particular had discouraged these interests, and both parents had strongly encouraged him into a career in medicine. Painting and music had become a sideline. While he was in college, he had drifted unthinkingly into medical school without really even considering what a life in medicine might be like. He flew through medical school; his almost photographic memory meant passing exams was a breeze. It was only when he hit residency and began working shifts in the ED that he suddenly realized he had made a poor career choice.

Although Asim had started his residency in a positive way, enthusiastic and engaged, he soon became disaffected, especially when he started having severe back pain that led to the diagnosis of ankylosing spondylitis, a painful arthritic back condition with no real cure. His back pain progressively became worse during his first year of residency, exacerbated by the inevitable physical maneuvers, sudden weight bearing, and changes of position that an ED doctor has to withstand in such a physically strenuous environment. To keep working effectively, he started taking narcotics to control the pain—in small doses initially, but rapidly increasing.

He found that, to make sure he could feed his habit, he had to make lifestyle changes. He had never had many girlfriends, but now he lost interest in females completely. He also lost interest in spending time with his residency colleagues at the hospital and had drifted to the outside of their social circle, with increasingly little involvement in residency activities. He quickly realized that if he volunteered to do elective rotations at other hospitals, he had more peace and less likelihood of being challenged by his colleagues or his training director. He started taking all of the away rotations he could, which of course only marginalized him further during his second year of residency.

At the end of this first consultation, because of his constant evasion and my impression that he was minimizing his drug use, I decided to insist on a drug screen being done immediately to see what exactly was in his body at that time. He became upset at this suggestion, accusing me of not believing him and saying that I was acting more like a police officer than a physician. Nevertheless, I insisted, and having phoned the pathology lab and informed the chief medical officer, I walked with him to ensure that he had the observed screening done immediately. Fortunately, as the chair of the hospital well-being committee, the medical staff bylaws gave me the authority to require a "for-cause" drug or alcohol screen on any physician suspected of being intoxicated at work.

As we walked over, we had a fascinating follow-up conversation.

"What drugs are you going to screen me for?" Asim asked diffidently. "Is this a screen for more than Oxycontin?"

"Yes, it certainly is," I responded. "The screens that I've ordered for you, and which will be done routinely, will pick up a wide range of both legal controlled substances, such as Oxycontin, and street drugs, such as meth, cocaine, and weed."

"Why are you doing that?" he replied. "After all, I've only taken Oxycontin."

"That's good, then," I said. "But you seem a bit worried about this drug screen, so if you've taken any other drugs, please tell me now so we can both know what the screen will show. The tests are very sensitive and will pick up an amazing range of drugs, remember."

"What about heroin?" he asked, to my almost complete surprise. I hadn't been expecting him to be taking an illegal narcotic when, as a doctor, getting hold of prescribed narcotics, especially in an ED, is relatively easy. "Will the test pick up heroin?"

"It certainly will, although as I'm sure you know, many people who think they've taken heroin end up taking other drugs that have been cut into whatever they bought. It sounds to me like you're saying that you think you've taken heroin. That's serious, as you know. How recently, and how has this happened?"

After completing the drug tests, Asim finally shared more of the story. It seemed that he had minimized his distress and drug usage dramatically. He now admitted to taking marijuana quite regularly at medical school as well as drinking excessively from college onward, with blackouts ending in a drunken stupor several times per year. He had managed to keep most of these events away from his parents because he was not living at home but was sharing an apartment with his elder brother, Samir, in whom he confided. Samir knew about Asim's drinking and drug use and was aware that he really wanted to study music and art rather than science; he had been trying to persuade Asim to see a counselor for several years. In Asim's final year of medical school, Samir had moved out of state to pursue his own career, leaving Asim without his primary support as he started residency.

Asim had chosen emergency medicine as his residency mainly because he felt it was the one specialty where, as a physician, you could turn up to do a shift of work, see your patients, and then go home. He hated the idea of worrying about any continuity of care and thought that this would not happen in the ED because others were always there to follow up behind you. As a medical student, he told me he had heard the term "lifestyle" specialties and thought that working in the ED, where he believed his work would be less consuming, would give him more of a chance to eventually get back to his art and music. He had not, however, realized just how difficult and personally traumatic working in an ED could be. Within a few months of starting residency, Asim was unable to sleep properly, was having nightmares of disturbed or dying patients, and could not rid his mind of the horrors that he witnessed. The final straw for him was having to try to save the life of a 22-year-old Indian woman who had set herself on fire in a bath of gasoline after her brand-new husband had been killed in a motor vehicle accident, in an ultimately successful attempt to join him in the afterlife. She had had 90% of her body covered in burns, and he had spent several minutes desperately trying to get a deep intravenous line going via her neck, one of the only unburned parts of her body. In the end he was successful, but all he could do was relieve her pain with morphine. She died within a few hours in the ED. He could not get the smell of burned flesh out of his brain, and for months afterward, whenever he smelled meat, he felt like vomiting. At work, when he saw sick individuals whom he was meant to save, he just wanted to run away and go home, sure he would fail. It was so unlike the rather naive and unrealistic perspective of the ED he had gained as a medical student, when he had been primarily an observer. By the end of his first year of residency, he had realized that he had made a mistake and should never have attempted to train in emergency medicine. He had phoned his brother to discuss his situation, feeling unable to talk to anyone else. The conversation had gone thus:

> Asim: "I need to talk to you about what I should do with myself, Samir. I have no one else I trust like you, and I wish you were here, even though I know you're doing what you want in your new job. I just wish you hadn't moved away. Perhaps I'll come out and spend a week with you when I get holidays in a few months. It would be good to get away from here."
>
> Samir: "I'm so sorry to hear that, Asim. I'd hoped things would get better for you over time and that you would settle into your work."
>
> Asim: "That's what I assumed, but it's not happening. We have to work so hard as residents, with usually just 1 day off per week and long

shifts. We never finish on time, because it takes a couple of hours to finish our notes at the end of each shift. We have no time to recover, and all I want to do is to sleep when I'm not at work. I never really enjoyed the work, as you know, but now I literally dread going in to the hospital. You wouldn't believe how some of the patients treat us, how hard it is to deal with them, and how much pressure is put on us by the senior medical staff and the nurses. We're just everyone's slaves, or so it feels like. "

Samir: "That sounds bad, indeed. Tell me more, I have lots of time."

Asim: "Well, two sets of issues worry me. First, I know I'm very burned out. I have all the classic features, and the degree of burnout we have seems to be the only thing my fellow residents want to talk about. But they're almost proud of it, as though they're surviving on the front line of a battle, whereas I hate it and feel hopeless and useless. I no longer see the point in trying to help patients; I just work them up as rapidly as possible so I can get home on time at the end of a shift. I keep thinking of walking out part way through a shift and just going home and spending a few hours painting. It sounds so good. But I can't do it."

Samir: "What's the second problem?"

Asim: "Well, that concerns one particular patient that I just cannot get out of my mind. I am constantly reminded of her. Whenever I smell burning, especially burned meat, I think of her and am taken back to what happened when she died. She seems to be all around me. Anything Indian or to do with the Hindu religion reminds me of her. If I pray, she's there. When I sleep, she's there. When I see anything violent on TV, she's there. The other day, I was walking down the street on my day off, and suddenly I went past a shop selling baths, with several in the window, and I thought I could see her sitting in one. I had a flashback to her being in the hospital, dying. It's so horrible. What can I do? The only thing that seems to help is drinking or taking a sedative to give myself some artificial sleep, so I've started to do that, but it worries me sometimes that I will be unable to get to work if I knock myself out too much. What should I do, Samir?"

Samir: "I am so sorry, Asim. I remember you mentioning this patient before, but I didn't realize you were so upset. What actually happened?"

Asim: "It wasn't just the horror of the situation. What upset me was the sort of person I think she was. She was beautiful and reminded me of an Indian version of our mom, from those pictures when she married Dad. She was wearing the remains of her wedding sari, a beautiful gown, now all burned and destroyed, and despite the massive pain of her burns, she still somehow looked at peace. She was only semiconscious, and when I tried to put a line into her neck to give her fluids and painkillers, she resisted, like she didn't want me to do it. She muttered something to me, and I had the impression she didn't want me to do anything to try to save her. I

ended up looking her in her eyes, upside down, as I eventually put
the line in her neck, and she seemed to be staring right through
me. I know she was looking at me as she finally became unconscious and died. I was the last person she saw. I think she was
pleased to see me, because she seemed to whisper something. I'm
not sure what it was, but I wonder if she was asking me to pray
for her. It was me pushing the morphine that ultimately killed her,
even though I know rationally that she could not possibly have
survived and that I was doing what my attending had told me to
do. But I did finally kill her, even though I took away her pain."

Samir: "I'm so sorry. I didn't realize you were having so much trouble.
Isn't there someone you can go and speak to about this?"

Asim: "Yes, there is, but it's too embarrassing, and I should be able to
manage this myself. All the other residents do. There's nothing
special about me; we all go through the same experiences, and we
all know we're doing a tough residency. The issue for me is how
best to cope and, perhaps more importantly, whether I should continue on or pull out and do something else. But what would Mom
and Dad say if I did that?"

Asim described how difficult each day at work became as the months
went by. He had symptoms of burnout that varied and were usually tol-
erable, but he had also developed chronic anxiety related to the posttraumatic stress disorder–like symptoms he had after the young Indian
woman's awful death and his part in it. He carried an unreasonable level
of guilt and was unable to talk about it and process his feelings. At the
same time, he had started having more chronic back pain from his arthritis, partly exacerbated by the physical work he had to do in the ED—lifting and rolling patients over to properly examine them and holding
flailing arms and legs down to help injured patients. He did finally find
a primary care physician and started taking painkillers on a regular basis,
which he often washed down with alcohol or with extra drugs he was
able to pocket during his daily work, such as sedatives and narcotics.
These were all too easy to obtain, either by just taking some from supplies
brought in by patients or from those given to patients as they left the department. When he was on night duty, with fewer nurses around to check
the medications, he could take them directly from the medication carts
themselves, signing them out in larger quantities than he gave to patients.

Asim knew that he was becoming an addict but rationalized his behavior by telling himself that he could always control his drug use if he
wanted, and could stop anytime, even if he seldom tried. By now he had
become a fairly isolated figure. He increasingly chose to do night and
weekend shifts where he could feed his addiction more easily and no
one seemed to care as long as he turned up and did his work. He man-

aged to continue in this way until the end of his second year of residency, when, much to his chagrin, he failed his annual exams. This led to an interview with his training director, Dr. Brucer, whom, up until that time, he had managed to avoid as much as possible:

> Dr. Brucer: "Asim, I'm surprised at you failing this recent exam. And I'm also concerned about you, because you seem to be pretty isolated, and the other residents tell me that you don't socialize with them at all. From my perspective, when we've been on shifts together, you seem at times to be rather withdrawn and anxious. Why do you think this is happening? Why did you fail the exam? It's not like you; you're usually near the top of your class."
>
> Asim: "I'm so sorry to disappoint you, Dr. Brucer. I know how much emphasis you put on our exam results and how important it is that we all pass so the comparison of our program with others is good. I'm so sorry to have let you down. I didn't mean to. I'm not sure what happened. There hasn't been anything unusual going on with me. I'm surprised by the things you say. My only issue is back pain, which you know about, and which has been a bit worse recently, as the letter to you from my primary care doc explained."
>
> Dr. Brucer (unconvinced, but trying to give him the benefit of the doubt): "Are you sure that's all, Asim? You do seem to have changed over the past 2 years. You used to smile more and took part in a lot of the resident team activities. I noticed you didn't attend the baseball and pizza night last week. I was sorry about that, because we had a great evening, and you were the only resident absent."
>
> Asim: "I know. I feel bad about that." [He had secretly planned to miss the evening by switching his shifts so he had to work at the time.] "It was unfortunate that I was scheduled to work at the time and couldn't get there. I'll try to switch my shifts for the next social to make sure I can come. I was trying to do a favor for Christine, who really wanted to go to the social. You know how upset she's been since her marriage broke up."
>
> Dr. Brucer: "All right. I guess you're right; we do always have to have coverage. And it was kind of you to cover for Christine. But what about the exams, Asim? I don't understand how you failed them so badly. When you're working, you always seem to have a good hold on the knowledge required. I know you gave me that letter about your back pain, but honestly, I've seen you on shifts in the department. You don't look like you have a lot of pain, so I'm not sure that's a full explanation."

Asim knew he had to deal with this issue and thought a lot about it. The reason for his poor performance had been simple; he had not done any extra work or study in the 2 weeks prior to the exams, like all the other residents did. He had been feeling particularly anxious, had not been sleeping, and had been taking more narcotics than usual, fooling himself constantly that he would get to his studying the next day. Unfortunately, the "next day" never came, and he ended up being unprepared for the exam and missing the revision sessions because he was too drugged up when not on work shifts. He'd thought that he could get out of the problem by getting a letter from his doctor explaining that he had more back pain than usual, but it seemed that this was not enough. As he was doing more and more often, he had decided to lie and make up excuses in the hope that Dr. Brucer would swallow his story, as she tended to do most of the time. He had long ago decided that he could deceive her fairly easily; she was so prepared to always believe the best and give the benefit of any doubt to "her" residents, whom at times she seemed to almost treat as her children. He had long since learned how lacking in curiosity or suspicion she was about his many explanations for aberrant behavior. So he had decided to give her a full house of reasons, both to elicit sympathy and avoid accountability. She was easy to fool, and he had become an expert at lying.

> Asim: "I really don't know what happened. I did the usual amount of study, but it just didn't seem to go in. I know it may seem odd to you, but my back pain is substantial, and it always seems to be worse when I'm in bed, so my sleep was disturbed. I also had a few phone calls from home, because my grandmother is sick, and my mom wanted my opinion on how to help her, even though this has been going on for ages, as you know. Perhaps all that together stopped me retaining what I was learning. If you remember, the ED was especially busy at the time, and I was on night shifts just before the exam, so I also didn't get to all the revision didactics. Maybe that all just accumulated and led to my poor performance. I know I have to take it again, and I wonder if I could take a few days' holiday before the next exam so that I can study properly. I'm really keen to show you what I can do."
>
> Dr. Brucer: "I'm so sorry, Asim. That really does sound difficult. I hadn't realized all those things were going on at once. Still, it's a shame that you failed, and you do have to repeat. I think your idea is a good one, and we'll work on schedules to arrange that next time. Thanks for your explanation."

Asim had managed to scrape past his exam a few weeks later by taking a week off work and focusing on doing as many practice tests as possible. For much of his third year of residency he managed to fly under the radar by doing just enough to pass any tests and quizzes and by being prepared to work antisocial hours, including weekends and holidays, to feed his now regular narcotic and tranquilizer habits. He knew he was seen as an outsider by his resident colleagues, but he didn't really care, because he hated his job. He thought that he had to complete his residency so as not to face humiliation from his parents and family, and he had vaguely started to wonder what he might do after he finished the 4-year program. He fantasized about taking an easy part-time job in an urgent-care clinic. That would allow him to return to his passions of art and music, which he had totally ignored during residency.

His life by then was completely controlled by his need for narcotics. Despite his internal denials, he had become thoroughly addicted, and most of his life was spent making sure he had a continuing supply of narcotics. He avoided Dr. Brucer as much as possible, which was not hard because she seldom did the night or weekend shifts for which he constantly volunteered. He had been surprised by how little interest was shown in him as long as he turned up and did passable work.

At the beginning of his third year, on a Saturday night shift, Dr. Chofan's situation took a major turn for the worse. He had run out of the Oxycontin he usually took to help him through his shift and was feeling on edge and somewhat irritable, consumed by the need to steal some narcotics during the next hour or so. Unfortunately, his addiction was recognized by a heroin-addicted patient he was examining. This patient was a regular "frequent flyer" in the ED, an elderly-looking 35-year-old man who called himself Duke. He had multiple medical problems as a result of his long-term heroin use and self-injecting, and he was also a dealer who lived close to Asim and recognized him.

When they were alone, Duke, who could almost smell a new client through long experience, asked Asim how he felt and told him he looked strung out. He had noted Dr. Chofan's subtle tremor, agitation, sweating, and pinpoint pupils, all signs of an addict in mild withdrawal. Asim initially had been both frightened and distressed at being confronted by a patient; if Duke could pick out his addiction so easily, surely others in the department might do so as well. How was it that they hadn't done so already? Duke spoke to him in a cunning, manipulative manner, promising a supply of heroin and any other drugs Asim wanted in the future while threatening to turn him in to the hospital authorities if Asim didn't give him his phone number and address, now that Duke knew his name. His well-practiced combination of promises and threats caused Dr. Chofan to panic and agree to meet with Duke the following day. One thing led to another, and Asim was soon buying heroin from Duke regularly, supplementing any drugs Asim continued to take at work. Asim had rationalized the situation as being less risky for himself because he no longer needed to steal so many narcotics at work, and he had decided to complete his final year of residency in whatever way he could, keeping his head down and avoiding his attendings and fellow residents as much as possible. Dr. Brucer eventually had enough, and several years later than she should have, she had insisted on referring him to me for assessment.

Asim gave up the pretense of just taking painkillers for his back, and after a long, difficult discussion, he agreed that I could arrange his immediate admission to a detox unit in an addiction center that had an inpatient addiction treatment program for professionals such as doctors, lawyers, and pilots.

So what happened next?

Fifteen years later, a much more mature and healthier-looking Asim told his story at a medical conference on addictions. In the interim period, he had spent 5 years in a diversion program, where he was treated for his addiction. During that time he also had qualified as an emergency medicine physician but found working in that specialty too difficult, even part-time, with the constant availability of drugs and the daily reminders of traumas and patient distress. After a few years, he ultimately realized he would not be commercially successful as an artist despite devoting a lot of time to it. He decided that he would continue working in medicine, but as a specialist in addiction medicine instead. It was in that role that he attended the addiction conference.

Asim looked out at the audience of about 300 physicians and started to tell his story.

"I am a narcotic addict," he began. "And I still struggle with my addiction every day, as I will for the rest of my life. The good news is that I have 15 years of sobriety behind me. I have faced my demons through individual therapy, medication management from a skilled physician, major lifestyle changes, long-term work with a group of physician and health care colleagues who attend Narcotics Anonymous, and the help and support of my family, many friends, and colleagues—my vital support network. I am still able to practice as a physician and have found an area of medicine that I love and that is truly rewarding. It's good to be a physician addict who is able to help other physician addicts as they move along their individual paths, usually with bumps in the road just as I had. I know I'm not cured, and never will be, because addiction is a lifelong disease. But I now look forward to the future with interest and excitement, knowing that I have a rewarding career path to follow. Medicine allows me to follow my other interests and pursuits while remaining a member of the medical profession, which has shown me remarkable tolerance and support. I am so proud to be a physician, and a recovering addict, who specializes in seeing other addicts, using both my medical and my personal knowledge and experiences to connect with my patients."

Asim looked out at the audience, who were engaged and listening carefully. He continued.

"But I am not here today to focus on my story. I am here to concentrate on solutions to the problem of physician addicts and to tell you what I have learned, good and bad, and what I believe needs to change so that future generations of physician addicts can be effectively and humanely treated and can continue to practice medicine and contribute to society in the way we all hoped to do on our first day of medical school."

Asim looked down at his notes. They were really just a guide for his talk; he had found that, as a result of doing a lot of public presentations, he was much more fluent and natural when he said what he felt rather than trying to be too formal. His notes read

> Focus on SOLUTIONS—not problems.
> BE POSITIVE.
> Changes that have helped me:
>
> - Acknowledging and learning to understand my chronic and lifelong disease
> - A caring, long-term addiction physician and my primary care physician
> - A supportive wife, family, and colleagues—my support network that is always available to me
> - Realizing I am not an imposter and am capable of being an excellent physician
> - A psychiatrist and health system that cared for me and had the means to get me into treatment
> - THE STRENGTH TO TELL PEOPLE ABOUT MY DISEASE
> - An emphasis on multimodal therapy, including buprenorphine and CONVENIENT, PRIVATE, AND RANDOM DRUG SCREENING
> - Narcotics Anonymous and group and individual therapy
> - Ability to keep working and maintain my medical license
> - Outside interests and passions
> - Time and patience
>
> Changes I would like to have made or seen:
>
> - MORE SLEEP AND EXERCISE; BETTER FOOD
> - Less STIGMA around addiction and mental health
> - Less fear of being found out (my parents know and have been great); less potential humiliation
> - More career preparation and planning in pre-med and med school—WHY did I go into medicine?
> - A more curious training director

- Colleagues who are trained to recognize illness in each other and take action as appropriate if others seem to be in trouble
- Education about self-care and physician well-being early on, with process groups to help us understand what we are going through—learning to engage with problems rather than avoid them so I would have been more resilient
- A changed culture of medicine where physician wellness is seen as essential; MORE SUPPORT FROM COLLEAGUES WHEN I WAS UNWELL
- Learning that acknowledging feelings and asking for help is OK
- Training for educators to identify students/residents in trouble, to pick us up early
- Easier ways of referring physicians to mental health professionals so we can obtain care

Asim looked up from his notes and addressed the audience again.

Commentary

Dr. Chofan's story is similar to those of thousands of doctors currently practicing medicine. His lecture notes are a good summary of the many positive solutions he found and the lifelong problems and barriers that such physicians report, as well as the best treatment approaches, as discussed in some detail in my previous book (Yellowlees 2018, Chapters 4 and 5). Here I focus on how to change the medical system and health industry to make such positive solutions and successful treatment more accessible.

Two issues of importance arise from this scenario. First is the culture of residency—what needs to change to make it more humane and more focused on self and communal care. This is starting to happen nationally, led by the Accreditation Council for Graduate Medical Education (2019) professionalism requirements for self-care, but we still have a long way to go. Second is the need for the availability of, and easy access to, good psychiatric and addiction treatment. Finally, because the prognosis of psychiatric and substance abuse treatment in physicians is generally good, with many physicians like Dr. Chofan being able to salvage their careers, greater understanding and better facilitation for these physicians to make directional changes in their careers are necessary. Although most doctors in the past have found a specialty and stayed with it for their entire careers, it is evident in our modern world that a number of doctors, for many reasons, will choose several perhaps very different medicine-related careers during their working lives. The entire health industry needs to adapt to facilitate this new reality.

Regarding the need for a culture of self-care, we know from a recent systematic review and meta-analysis of 54 studies involving 17,560 physicians in training (Mata et al. 2015) that, overall, 28% of trainees screened positive for depression during residency and that resident burnout levels are twice those of age-matched control subjects after controlling for work hours. In terms of solutions to this major problem, which can no longer be denied, Margaret Rea, Ph.D., director of resident well-being at University of California (UC), Davis, has made the point that although systems issues and stressors need to be a primary focus, it is important to know how and when to offer support and resources for students and trainees. She noted that maintaining well-being needs to be part of the developing identity of every health care professional if we are to change the landscape about physician well-being (University of California, Davis Health 2019).

Residents as a group are known to exhibit the following set of pre-existing psychological strengths and vulnerabilities, as shown in the scenario: high internal pressure to succeed, commitment, caring, perfectionism, self-criticism and self-doubt, fear of making mistakes, self-deprecation, compassion fatigue, compulsiveness, feelings of inferiority, and the common belief that somehow they are an impostor and do not deserve their new role as a physician. Krasner et al. (2019) demonstrated similar attitudes in primary care physicians. When the many external environmental causes affecting residents, such as an overwhelming workload, looming debt, high external expectations of success and perfection, competitiveness, lack of community, a culture that does not allow for vulnerability, a lack of control, and the stigma around mental health treatment are added to the burden, it is hardly surprising that it is difficult to engage residents in care. I remember one resident recently who told me it took a month to find time to have a much-needed haircut, which is a much easier task than engaging in care.

We know that most medical students and residents who are depressed or suicidal do not seek formal help. Indeed, it took Dr. Chofan a great deal of time and encouragement to do so. Numerous studies have examined why this is, and Dr. Rea has summarized the reasons as lack of time, concerns about confidentiality, worry about cost, fear of documentation on academic records or licensing boards, fear of losing the respect of their colleagues if their depression became public, and concern that faculty would view them as unfit for their responsibilities (University of California, Davis Health 2019).

What, then, are the solutions for residents? Dr. Chofan noted some in his lecture notes, such as the need for multiple approaches to well-being to change the culture of residency for future generations of doctors. Dr. Rea has described these many approaches as they occur at UC Davis, which has a formal office of wellness and a multimodal resident well-being program. The approaches include, among others, a resident wellness committee, a newsletter, workshops, process groups and debriefings, mentoring, access to a self-assessment mental health survey (Haskins et al. 2016), and easy 24/7 access to confidential counseling and psychiatric services, especially during work hours (University of California, Davis Health 2019). Education on burnout, depression, substance use, sleep hygiene, mindfulness, team dynamics, exercise, communication skills, and relationships is also available. Other solutions are described in the many popular books about "surviving residency" for residents themselves (Peterkin 2016) or for residents' partners (Math 2008) or that humanize the life of physicians (Elton 2018). Elton (2018) placed a strong focus on the importance of the transitions from medical student to resident and from resident to attending, noting the importance of students having supervised time and practice in these new roles before taking on full responsibilities. Most medical schools now include "mini-internships" that medical students can take in their last year, as well as acting-attending roles for residents to take, typically in their last year of residency, and these are to be encouraged. This changing culture is very different from the traditional approach to new skills development taught historically in medicine—that is, "see one, do one, teach one"—as I was taught throughout my early career.

The second focus in this chapter is the need for residents to receive good psychiatric and addiction treatment, just as Dr. Chofan received. The physician as patient was addressed by Myers and Gabbard (2008) in a comprehensive clinical handbook focused on treatment by mental health professionals. Unfortunately, despite this, physicians still frequently receive second-class care for many reasons (Yellowlees 2018), including their own failure to recognize their needs, the stigma surrounding mental health, and providers' inabilities to deliver high-quality care to VIPs—whom I noted (Yellowlees 2018) could be considered either "very important" or "very intimidating" patients. Psychiatrists, as the obvious highly trained professional group capable of delivering such care to their colleagues, should be more proactively involved in delivering and promoting this treatment than they are at present and should collaborate with addiction specialists as appropriate (Nakagawa and Yellowlees 2019). At present, most cities have a professional network that guides physicians in need of mental health treatment to a few specialists (usually psychiatrists, psychologists, and addiction specialists) who over time have become the local experts, but not everyone knows how to access such informal networks. This ultimately becomes yet another barrier to physicians who need care. Although physicians receive specialized medical training, their knowledge and expertise do not necessarily enable them to maintain their own personal wellness or model best practices for themselves.

Psychiatrists are in a unique position to serve as the "physician's physician" in various roles. Most physicians receive very limited training in psychiatry and do not have the skills and knowledge to detect early signs of burnout, depression, addiction, and suicidal thoughts and behaviors in their colleagues or in themselves. This lack of formal training and experience makes it hard for many physicians to take proactive steps to speak to a colleague in distress, perhaps through fear of professional repercussions or of damaging relationships. This places psychiatrists in prime position to help their organizations raise awareness and develop effective prevention, detection, and management programs. Historically, psychiatrists have not been proactive enough in promoting the relevance of their skills to helping colleagues and organizations tackle this hidden epidemic.

The first role for psychiatrists as the "physician's physician" is as a clinician-educator, for many reasons. As Nakagawa and Yellowlees (2019) described, physicians may be challenging to treat as patients. Overidentification, intimidation, and politics can negatively influence care for the impaired physician, which may lead to deviations from the standard of care that other patients would have received (Yellowlees 2018). Physician patients commonly influence or dictate their own treatment plans, which leads to a tendency to deviate from standard treatment approaches (Alfandre et al. 2016), such as excluding physical examinations; delaying drug screens, which Dr. Chofan noted were important for his continued sobriety; and ignoring the role of the primary care physician.

Treating physicians may also have difficulty being honest with their physician patients or may appease or inappropriately go along with patients' unusual demands, with both parties potentially losing clinical objectivity. Another major concern is protecting the privacy of physician patients, who will likely be sensitive about being seen in waiting rooms, so it is not uncommon for appointments to be scheduled outside of regular clinic hours or to occur in unusual places, such as their homes. Physician patients often prefer to be referred outside of their practice networks and may pay cash to avoid their employers or insurers having any record of their visits, whereas other physician patients tend to expect priority treatment, such as being able to call the treating physician's cell phone directly. It may be helpful to offer all of these approaches, but it is critical to set clear limits.

As part of this direct treatment role, within a health system or clinical network, psychiatrists can help support and identify colleagues at risk for depression, burnout, and suicide. They can create an informal referral network that includes a psychiatrist who is available to provide information and anonymous curbside or supportive consultations as well as education on well-being for all physicians. An understanding colleague can be just one phone call away. One key educational intervention is to teach about the difference between having a disorder, such as depression or multiple sclerosis, and a disability or an impairment. The latter may cause work-related difficulties and require reporting through appropriate internal or external channels, potentially ultimately to a physician health program or occasionally directly to medical boards. Most physician patients with a psychiatric or substance-related problem have an illness but are not likely impaired for work in any functional way. They should be treated clinically and reassured that no reporting is necessary, especially, as discussed in Chapter 2, because most medical boards are moving away from concern over diagnoses toward focusing on current impairment when considering individual capacity for physicians to practice medicine.

The other key role for psychiatrists is to be an administrative physician leader. Psychiatrists are well placed to play an instrumental role in driving the culture of physician well-being for their organizations. This is an opportunity for psychiatrists to help craft policies and guidelines as well as serve as valuable leaders and contributors to every organization by serving as chief wellness officer (see Chapter 2), chairing or being a member of a physician well-being committee, or working with a statewide physician health program (Yellowlees 2018, Chapter 9). These roles also offer opportunities for professional development and career enrichment for psychiatrists looking to expand the scope of their practice, engage in physician leadership, and leverage their clinical expertise to shape policies at the local and national levels (Nakagawa and Yellowlees 2019).

The third role for psychiatrists is to collaboratively lead the medical profession into the future. The country's health care workforce is rapidly changing, with a new generation of physicians entering clinical practice and the Baby Boomer generation of physicians set to retire. Technologies such as telemedicine and smartphones are enabling more flexible and mobile work arrangements. Yellowlees and Shore (2018) described how psychiatrists can become hybrid practitioners delivering digital treatments, discussed later in Chapter 8, which may well suit physician patients excellently by allowing them to increasingly be treated privately and potentially at home. Psychiatrists can lead the way by adapting to these new changes and evolving their practices accordingly. Today's culture and work environments need to change rapidly to support the values and work-life equilibria sought by the Millennial generation, and these changes will also be in synchrony with the needs of physicians. It is likely that in the not too distant future, a physician treatment network will develop like those available for other demographic, racial, or diagnostic groups, and psychiatrists should lead such a network. The changes in residency applications to various specialties are indicators of the shift in workforce preferences, with increasing applications to lifestyle specialties such as dermatology, emergency medicine, and, in recent years, to psychiatry at the expense of disciplines such as surgery, which cannot currently fill its residency slots. Although Millennials are often described as "high maintenance" or "entitled," they are also known to prioritize family, friends, and hobbies, making them more resilient to burnout and better at self-care than previous generations of doctors. Physicians from other generations need to learn from their younger colleagues (Hershatter and Epstein 2010; Landrum 2018).

Psychiatrists need to be open to opportunities to lead and support physician health in communities and should lead by example as individuals and as a specialty, modeling self and collegial care to other professional groups within medicine. Nakagawa and Yellowlees (2019) noted that it is during residency that psychiatrists learn the professional demands of clinical practice, and this is a critical time to teach best practices on wellness and self-care to all psychiatric residents. Psychiatrists' everyday actions and behaviors can then have more impact on their colleagues and health systems and should elevate their profession's visibility and impact at the organizational and national levels. The country's health care spending is on an unsustainable trajectory, while the physician shortage problem will only get worse as more physicians retire. Lost productivity due to physician burnout, depression, and addiction is no longer just a physician wellness issue; it has become a national policy issue. For the health care system to gain more value out of every health care dollar, maintaining a healthy, productive physician workforce is absolutely critical. By forcefully promoting themselves as the "physician's physician," psychiatrists can contribute greatly to the wider health care system.

References

Accreditation Council on Graduate Medical Education: Improving Physician Well-Being, Restoring Meaning in Medicine (website). Chicago, IL, Accreditation Council on Graduate Medical Education, 2019. Available at: https://www.acgme.org/What-We-Do/Initiatives/Physician-Well-Being. Accessed May 9, 2018.

Alfandre D, Clever S, Farber NJ, et al: Caring for 'very important patients'—ethical dilemmas and suggestions for practical management. Am J Med 129(2):143–147, 2016 26522793

Elton C: Also Human: the Inner Lives of Doctors. New York, Basic Books, 2018

Haskins J, Carson JG, Chang CH, et al: The suicide prevention, depression awareness and clinical engagement program for faculty and residents at the University of California Davis Health System. Acad Psychiatry 40(1):23–29, 2016

Hershatter A, Epstein M: Millennials and the world of work: an organization and management perspective. J Bus Psychol 25(2):211–223, 2010

Krasner MS, Epstein RM, Beckman H, et al: Association of an educational program in mindful communication with burnout, empathy, and attitudes among primary care physicians. JAMA 302(12):1284–1293, 2009 19773563

Landrum S: Millennials to be the most high-maintenance in the workplace. Forbes, January 12, 2018. Available at: https://www.forbes.com/sites/sarahlandrum/2018/01/12/millennials-to-be-the-most-high-maintenance-in-the-workplace. Accessed May 10, 2019.

Mata DA, Ramos MA, Bansal N, et al: Prevalence of depression and depressive symptoms among resident physicians: a systematic review and meta-analysis. JAMA 314(22):2373–2383, 2015 26647259

Math K: Surviving Residency: A Medical Spouse Guide to Embracing the Training Years. Sartell, MN, C and B Press, 2008

Myers M, Gabbard GO. The Physician as Patient: A Clinical Handbook for Mental Health Professionals. Washington, DC, American Psychiatric Publishing, 2008

Nakagawa K, Yellowlees P: The physician's physician: the role of the psychiatrist in helping other physicians and in promoting wellness. Psychiatr Clin North Am 42(3):473–482, 2019

Peterkin A: Staying Human During Residency Training: How to Survive and Thrive After Medical School, 6th Edition. Toronto, ON, University of Toronto Press, 2016

University of California, Davis Health: Graduate Medical Education Wellness Program (website). Sacramento, CA, University of California, Davis, 2019. Available at: https://health.ucdavis.edu/gme/wellness.html. Accessed May 9, 2019.

Yellowlees P: Physician Suicide: Cases and Commentaries. Washington, DC, American Psychiatric Association Publishing, 2018

Yellowlees P, Shore J (eds): Telepsychiatry and Health Technologies: A Guide for Mental Health Professionals. Washington, DC, American Psychiatric Association Publishing, 2018

Chapter 8

COGNITIVE DISSONANCE AND DEFINING MEANING IN MEDICINE

Scenario

Christina Alfonso looked across the candlelit dinner table at her childhood sweetheart and husband, Roberto, as he gesticulated animatedly to illustrate a key point in his conversation. He was a handsome man. Roberto had pulled out all the stops tonight—new beige sport coat and an open-neck, bright white shirt that showed off his strong, classically Hispanic features and jet-black hair. She thought to herself how much she loved him and how lucky they were to have been able to make their life work together so successfully. She was pleased she had dressed up tonight; she had loved hearing Roberto tell her how beautiful she looked in the car on the way to the restaurant. Her long, dark hair showed off her ivory complexion and dark brown eyes. She was wearing the black cocktail dress Roberto had surprised her with earlier that day and her grandmother's antique gold necklace and earrings.

The restaurant lights in the upmarket Mexican restaurant in Southern California were dim, punctuated by multiple carefully lit fountains of colored water that played over the wine bottle displays hanging from the walls and cascaded down to the floor. Despite the many noisy groups of diners and constant clashing of plates and cutlery from the busy serving staff, the four close friends, seated at a corner table away from the bar, were able to hear each other easily.

Roberto had just been describing his latest architectural success, a carbon-neutral luxury resort he and his team had designed on the Baja coast. A partner in an international group of architects, Roberto was usually the point man on such projects, which meant going to, and living at, the locations while they were constructed, working with local builders, and supervising the construction of a range of increasingly large and sophisticated building complexes. His hands whirled like out-of-control windmills as he demonstrated how he had finished off the massive entertainment complex by incorporating a solid rock face as one wall, a masterpiece of art and engineering as well as a huge energy saver in a hot climate. Christina had heard this story before and was happy to only half listen as she thought about their life together and how lucky they were. Their friends at the table, Jose and Alexia, were both family medicine physicians who had been classmates of Christina's at medical school. Jose had given up trying to interrupt the almost-unstoppable Roberto, but Alexia was successful at last after playfully grabbing Roberto's hand and pulling it back down to earth to halt his torrent of excitable explanations.

"Roberto. We know you love your architecture, but why can't you just show us some pictures? Your hands are very mobile, and your voice descriptive, but it's hard to visualize a multipurpose entertainment complex in a cave," she said.

"Of course," Roberto laughed. "Here, let me show you on my phone. I have hundreds of photos; let me find the best ones for you." He pulled out his smartphone and tapped on the photo icon immediately, bringing up several dramatic photos of his work.

"Wow. That's cool, Roberto," said Jose. "The walls facing away from the rock face remind me a bit of that building you designed a couple of years ago in Santiago. You know the one I mean. You had a whole series of eels featured throughout the building as a theme, because they are such a delicacy in Chile. Wasn't that the building you got the big architectural award for?"

"Yes, you're right. I always try to bring in a local theme or important set of cultural beliefs whenever I build a major complex, but I combine that with making sure the complex is as energy efficient as possible. You know how important combating climate change is to both Christina and me. In Baja, you see those tall, red figures that look like they emerged from the cave. They're meant to remind you of the ancient rock paintings, hieroglyphs and pictographs, painted all over the Baja Peninsula by indigenous people in the prehistoric age. Those paintings were included on the World Heritage list in the 1990s, so it's hard for visitors to see the magnificent artwork of the ancients unless they have an official guide. Now, they can visit this beautiful resort and experience the feel of these amazing 30-foot-high motifs for themselves, just as Christina and I did when we traveled the peninsula while I researched which figures would fit the hotel environment best. The big difference, though, is that in the resort they can keep cool without damaging the planet!"

Alexia took Roberto's phone and started flicking through his photos. Spain, Italy, Morocco, Canada, and Australia all appeared in rapid succession. Many photos included Christina and their two sons, now aged 4 and 6 years.

"I can't believe how many countries you've worked in during the past few years. What an amazing array! It's no surprise we only see you here occasionally, with all these trips," Alexia said. "Our kids are only slightly younger than yours, and we're constantly rushing to keep up with their needs and our work. It seems as though we never get a break, except when we come out to dinner with you guys to find out about your most recent travels. How do you do it? Especially you, Christina. You're a physician, like us. I would love to know more about your virtual practice. You've never really told us a lot about it, but I looked up your website earlier today and have some understanding of what you do. I must say, it looks very interesting. I didn't realize you had so many colleagues involved. Can you tell us some more about it?"

Christina looked gratefully across the table at her friend, thanking her inwardly for giving her an insert into the conversation and for diverting Roberto, who could have continued with his dramatic stories for hours yet, and probably would, later. As she prepared to respond, however, Roberto interrupted enthusiastically.

"She's amazing, my wife. See how beautiful she is! She is my dream girl and 10 times more intelligent than me. She manages to work with patients all over the U.S. while she travels with me around the world, and she still manages our boys! All I do is spend time yelling at local builders and negotiating with owners who want to spend as little as possible while building as much as possible. I can't understand how she does it. She's a miracle worker. I love her."

"Now, Roberto. That's enough," Christina chided him gently. "It's my turn to talk. Let me get in and explain what I do." She gave him a look that was a combination of love and steely determination, which he well understood as denoting his time to take a back seat and control his energy.

"I'm glad you looked at our website, Alexia. Did you see it also, Jose? Or did Alexia explain much about it to you?"

"She mentioned it in the car, but she didn't go into a lot of detail. Of course, you talked about it a bit when we last met a year ago, but it was all in the early stages then," said Jose. "Why don't you just fill us in properly? We're both eager to hear about it and rather jealous of what you've done, living this amazing international lifestyle you have through Roberto's work. We're constantly stressed and only managed a short holiday to the Grand Canyon this year, yet you've been working in several countries, and you both look remarkably well and relaxed. How do you do it?"

"Well, it's no great secret. I mainly work as a virtual physician coach, which I can do from anywhere with broadband. I love what I'm doing and really feel I'm making a difference. It's so meaningful. I get to use many of the communication and planning skills that I learned in our internal medicine training, but on top of that I've gotten my MBA[1] and qualified as an executive coach over the past few years—all through online courses and mentoring, with occasional in-person retreats. I was doing reasonably well up until about a year ago, mainly with individual physician clients whom I would see regularly on videoconferencing. The physicians I helped were generally self-referred and were often burned out and at the end of their tether, so it was a hard process getting enough individual referrals to keep me busy. Physicians are just so reticent to get help for themselves, as I'm sure you both know. Why, I used to spend as much time finding clients as I did helping them! It was almost like trying to develop a private practice that consisted only of patients who either really didn't want to see you or were ashamed that it was necessary. There's still so much stigma over counseling for anything related to mental health."

"So what changed?" asked Alexia.

"What changed is that I had forgotten that medicine is a team sport and that we live in a rapidly changing world," Christina said, smiling. "It's really very obvious when you think about it. What I did was connect

---

[1]MBA=Master of Business Administration.

with a range of colleagues to form a virtual group consulting practice. We have several doctors, some behavioral health experts and psychiatrists, one addiction specialist, and a few lifestyle and strategic-planning consultants. This level of expertise is so much more than any one of us could achieve individually. Instead of taking on individual physicians as clients, although we still do that sometimes, we now consult to large health systems around the world and take a systemic and organizational view toward changing their cultures and their future planning. It's so much more interesting, and I've been able to incorporate my long-standing interest in climate change as well, because so many health systems are now trying to be more carbon focused."

"Hmm, I can see how that must feel rewarding, and why you need such a wide range of skills and expertise," Alexia said. "But why now? I can't imagine my clinic having the level of interest to bring you in. I suspect you must be very expensive—" She laughed. "Certainly judging by the quality of your jewelry tonight!"

Christina smiled and explained the jewelry had been inherited long ago from her grandmother. After a few minutes, she returned to the story of her business.

"All the recent work on physician burnout and the implications of that in terms of cost and quality has really made CEOs[2] around America sit up and think. This is the hot topic of the moment. Have you noticed how many articles on burnout and physician well-being are appearing in the medical journals? I've heard colleagues talk about how physicians are suddenly being seen as the equivalent of canaries in a coal mine; they're the first group showing symptoms as a reflection of the underlying stress on the whole current health care system. Is this not something you are hearing?"

"Yes, it is. You're right," said Jose. "Attitudes are changing toward the whole topic of physician well-being. We had a grand rounds presentation on the topic of burnout a few weeks ago. I've never seen such a well-attended presentation. The whole room was full to overflowing, and the presenter was inundated with questions afterward. Several of our physicians talked openly about how burned out they felt. I've always thought a lot of stigma was attached to admitting symptoms of burnout, but that seems to have almost gone now. It was actually a very interesting lecture. The main point made was that physicians should not be blamed as the cause of their burnout because they are somehow

---

[2]CEOs=chief executive officers.

weak. Instead, the lecturer showed evidence that most physicians are actually very resilient people who are simply working in a crazy, unreasonable system that doesn't allow them to perform. He showed data that upon entry to medical school students are less burned out than other postgraduate students, but 10 years into practicing they're twice as burned out as nonmedical professionals. It was compelling and made perfect sense to me. Also, it was something I'd read about previously. It was clearly good news for much of the audience; why, one of the surgeons, during the question section, openly thanked the lecturer for being the first person he'd ever heard who didn't blame physicians for getting burned out through lack of moral strength or resilience. The presenter received a massive round of applause from the audience, and we all talked about the lecture among ourselves afterward. I suspect there'll be some active follow up and, I hope, some action, although I'm not sure what will happen or help."

Christina laughed. "Well, that's why you need to contact us, Jose! Your story is typical of many health groups around the country. They've started to hear about this problem of burnout and lack of physician well-being. Some even call burnout a moral problem rather than a health problem. I'm actually quite sympathetic toward that view. And when you combine that with the threat of climate change, and how many of our current health practices are actually harming us through excess carbon emissions, the argument for change is compelling."

"What do you mean by a moral problem?" said Alexia. "Surely burnout is a set of symptoms, like a syndrome, if not a full diagnosis?"

"Well, the people who talk about a moral problem point to the fact that almost all students, when they enter medical school, do so because they want to spend lots of time with patients, have therapeutic relationships, and cure people. Nowadays, with the excessive amount of administrative work needed in American medicine, most physicians spend more time doing nonpatient work for billing and administration while using electronic records. Burnout is seen as a moral problem because it's an indication that physicians are not allowed sufficient time to do their jobs properly, or in the way that they want. That raises the moral question of whether they should continue this way, which leads to the symptoms that we recognize as burnout. It actually makes a lot of sense to me."

Christina saw Alexia nod in comprehension, and then she went on. "Although most physicians have read about the size of the burnout problem, how up to 50% of physicians have at least one of the three major symptoms or behavioral components of burnout, what no one really knows is what the solution, or solutions, are. The market is rapidly expanding for groups like mine that can refocus whole health systems, and hundreds of physicians and other key providers, to work more efficiently, effectively, and happily. What we do is present a range of possible solutions. We try to make self-care, and the care of colleagues, core aims of a changed health care culture. If necessary, we can coach or provide psychiatric treatment for individual physicians within the system using our team of experts spread all over the world. Climate change is surprisingly similar, so we usually include some simple advice on carbon-saving strategies. After all, no medical student entered medicine intending to make the world a less healthy place to live in as an unintended consequence of providing care. So, as a consulting group, we aim to make clinician well-being and carbon neutrality strategic aims of the organizations we work with, aims that are just as important as quality of patient care. We go into organizations—we have both in-person and online consultants—and learn how to better support their physicians as the core individuals driving quality and patient safety. This increases physician retention and reduces the costs of impaired patient care. That's why we need a multidisciplinary consulting team."

"See, I told you, my wife is a genius!" exclaimed Roberto, who was feeling rather left out of the conversation as the only nonphysician at the table. "Christina is always looking forward. She's a builder, just like I am, only she builds teams and organizations in a healthy way, whereas I stick to bricks and mortar. And she does it while still looking after our family, wherever we happen to be living at the time. Let's all toast Christina, and all the technologies she uses to help her professional colleagues!" Roberto raised his glass and clinked it with those of his wife and two friends. "You know what? Why don't you tell Alexia and Jose that story you told me last week about the work you've been doing in New York over the past year? Some of the feedback you've been getting is phenomenal, and from what you said, has already led to you being asked to help a number of other health systems."

Christina looked at her husband doubtfully. "I'm not sure Alexia and Jose really want to hear that much about my work over dinner. I thought we were here for a pleasant social evening, not a work-dominated meetup."

"Actually, we'd love to know how you do it, Christina," said Jose. "We're both fascinated by how you manage to maintain a professional lifestyle, using your medical training, while at the same time living all around the world, and seemingly without major stress on your family. We'd love to know how to do that."

"Jose is right, Christina," Alexia agreed. "We've been looking seriously at resigning from our current jobs and both feel quite burned out at times, but we haven't yet found a good alternative, so we stay where we are because we really like our patient panels and just hope our environment will improve over time. Finding out how you do this is of real interest to us."

"I'm so sorry to hear that, Alexia; I hadn't realized you were having such difficulty at work." Christina paused. "Well, if you want to hear what I do, let me tell you." She looked around the restaurant and nodded at a passing waiter, asking him to bring more sparkling water. Then she began to explain.

"When we start a contract, one or more of the company's principal consultants goes and spends a week or two with the health system to get to know it in some detail and to examine its data systems. I tend to do most of my work remotely; I rarely go to the health system in person. The EMRs[3] of course contain a lot of data sources, such as time logged, unfinished notes, and numbers of inbox messages, and many other sources can be found on the dashboards that many hospitals keep nowadays, including clinical and operational data. We are particularly interested in patient complaints and staff incident reports, especially those describing possible behavioral problems in physicians, because these are often a marker of high levels of burnout and systemic dysfunction. Then I look at the data on sick days, holidays not taken, physician turnover, numbers of legal suits, satisfaction surveys from patients and staff, and even the system's social media presence. It's fascinating. Increasingly, our clients already have gathered specific data from one of the many burnout surveys available, and their surprise at the results of those surveys is sometimes what leads to us being called in. After all, you can hardly do a burnout survey and not offer some sort of intervention when you find high levels of burnout!"

Christina took a sip of her water before continuing. "We look at the data and any other relevant information and interview key physicians and other senior managers. It's a bit like a root cause analysis. The aim then is to define the solutions most likely to be effective for whatever is happening, and that is the series of interventions we propose. Most of my work is carried out online, in collaboration with the health system, although we always have an in-person consultant working locally. We use a model that's very similar to that of the EMR companies. You know

---

[3]EMRs=electronic medical records.

how they typically charge a certain amount for their software and consulting but always insist that health systems employ their own IT[4] teams to do most of the implementation, support, training, and local management?" Her friends nodded. "Most health systems know that the cost of an EMR to the hospital is usually, at most, half of the total cost once all the mandated internal costs are taken into account. It's a clever model because everyone has skin in the game—the EMR company gets paid for a carefully identified scope of work, and the buying health system, although they usually underestimate how much their costs will be, cannot get away without sustaining them if they want to manage the EMR independently. So we do the same. We provide in-person and online expertise and consulting, the latter of which I do, but we insist that the health system pay some of their own staff to work with us while we actually implement solutions and change over time. The big advantage is that, like the EMR, the health system owns the change process and can continue on without us after our contract is finished. Or, of course, they can invite us back to do more consulting!" Christina chuckled. "Now that we've been doing our consulting for a while, we're in a position where we don't need to go out hunting for work. The need for what we do is so great that we now get most of our referrals by word of mouth."

"That's a clever financial model, I must say, and the partnership approach you take must be interesting. I see how you can do all this online using that model, but what sorts of interventions do you suggest?" Alexia asked. "Most of us know what the problems are, we just can't work out how to find an effective solution."

"Well, the solutions vary, of course, but we've become experts in some that almost always provide significant early gains and an early win. We focus carefully on how the system uses the EMR, which EMR they have, and their process for training their providers on the EMR, to see how efficiently they use the software itself. We also examine how much time the physicians are spending on the EMR, especially pajama time at home in the evenings and weekends, to see how efficiently—or otherwise—they are using it. You'd be amazed by how many physicians spend upward of a dozen hours per week catching up on their notes and inboxes at home! We also examine what clinical payer contracts the health system has, because it's the payers' requirements for billing and data collection that often lead to physicians doing excessive documentation, much more than is needed for normal clinical notes."

---

[4]IT = information technology.

"Why all that disparate data?" said Jose. "I get that most of us use the EMR badly and would love to have more time to spend with our patients. I read one paper last week describing a time and motion study that observed doctors at work; it showed that they spent more time on the EMR each day than actually talking to patients. I know that's what I do some days. It's so frustrating, and I feel so out of control. What do you do with the data?"

"Good question, Jose. This is where our consulting company has its 'secret sauce,' so to speak. We usually focus on two things as our early intervention, and between them they reduce the amount of physicians' screen time on the EMR by as much as 10%–20%. That gives them way more time to spend with their patients or, preferably, with their spouses and children. At the same time, we suggest some easy, quick changes they can make to save carbon emissions, which is always popular with physicians in particular."

"You're making us drag it out of you!" laughed Alexia. "What on Earth can you do to get results like that? Training us to use the software better would make a difference, I'm sure, but not that much. And if you can make that sort of change, why isn't every health system in the country doing the same?"

Christina was pleased at the obvious interest being shown by her friends. "Well, you mentioned training. Let me ask both of you—you use an EMR, which is a highly complicated and sophisticated piece of software. How much training have you actually had on it?"

Alexia responded first. "When the EMR was introduced a few years ago, we had 2 days of training and then access to some super-users who taught us shortcuts for a few months. Mostly, we taught ourselves. I usually look around for the youngest physicians I can find, often the residents, and ask them for help when I'm stuck. They seem to manage the supposedly intuitive parts of the EMR better than those of us who were brought up on paper records."

"So how much regular training do you get now?" Christina asked. "And what happens when your EMR is upgraded, as they are most years? Do you get any extra training?"

"We try to plan our holidays for those times," laughed Jose. "It's always impossible. Everything changes, and we just get sent a list of apparent improvements along with complicated screen shots showing how to access them. I know the help desk gets a lot more calls after an upgrade, and we take a lot longer writing our notes in the first few days while we explore the changes and figure out what the EMR does now and how that differs from the previous version. It's crazy, but I guess we're all just used to it and accept the process. The last time that happened, it took me more than a month to really work out properly how to prescribe online, and I must have wasted 10–15 hours using my own workarounds, which, in retrospect, were very ineffective. The good news is that I have learned that physicians are superb at finding workarounds, but I really wish someone could have just told me in the first place how to prescribe using two-factor identification on my phone."

"I'm so sorry, Jose," Christina responded. "That sounds frustrating. But what you're describing is the norm for most physicians around the country. For some reason, training on how to use the EMR efficiently so that it fits into your workflow, and not the other way around, is simply not common. You spent years and years learning the pharmacology of drugs, with constant updates, but are given almost no time to learn how to prescribe them electronically, which with today's narcotic epidemic is becoming much more complicated. My company implements regular one-on-one training for physicians on how to effectively use the EMR in their own clinical environment. It's complicated, because different physicians have different uses for the EMR and, therefore, different training needs. Compare yourself as a primary care physician with an emergency medicine or inpatient doc. You need access to very different sets of information and colleagues, and the way you document is also different. So training has to be individualized to a great extent, and we have to convince our clients, the CEOs, that this relatively expensive training approach makes financial sense. Return on investment still rules their brains. Fortunately, we can now do that reasonably easily, but we have to use their own data to convince them. Hence the need for data."

"Can you believe that my physician wife uses more math skills than I do as an engineer and architect?" said Roberto, keen to keep himself involved in the conversation somehow. "It's taken me a while to get used to seeing her poring over large spreadsheets of numbers so she can convert them into language that proves the need for the changes she is proposing. I always used to think I was the math expert in the house, but I'm now outdone."

"The training makes sense, but what about the issue of extra documentation that you mentioned? How can that be changed?" said Alexia. "This is becoming a hot issue for physicians around the country. I imagine you've read the recent article that compared documentation in the clinical notes of physicians in the U.S., Australia, and Europe; we reviewed it at our last case conference. The results were amazing! U.S. physicians wrote at least three times more than doctors in the other countries, yet we really don't work differently. That's why I feel like a data-entry clerk much of the time, and it's a reflection on the amount of administrative pressure put on us to collect data for billing and reporting."

"You got it in one, Alexia!" said Christina. "We spend a lot of time working with the health systems and their physicians, usually via video, and that's the part of the job I specialize in—reviewing this issue with them. We also make it clear that, if they copy us and use more video visits for meetings and with patients, that that also saves gas with less traveling. In our company, we are fanatical about actually trying *not* to fly for work, so most of the traveling I do is related to our home life and Roberto's jobs around the world. With our clients, we have to negotiate with the funders and payors, of course, to determine the minimum amount of documentation required for their administrative or billing purposes, and we work with the IT and coding teams, but once we've been given the go-ahead to reduce unnecessary documentation, we can usually cut it down markedly. I often end up having a lot of individual sessions with physicians, during which I essentially give them permission to write less and not just replicate large parts of their notes from visit to visit. All that duplication makes notes very hard to review rapidly. I've learned a lot about physicians through this consulting and how, as a profession, we are inherently good people. One of the harder parts of this problem is that often the physicians themselves are so afraid of doing the wrong thing, of perhaps being accused of billing fraud, that they tend to go overboard and write way too much rather than just enough. Of course, we all hear of occasional colleagues who are jailed for awful, fraudulent behavior, which drives this fear more, but the reality is that almost all physicians are good, honest people who write too much because they're afraid of not writing enough. It's crazy, when you think of it."

"That's a really interesting insight, Christina," said Alexia. "I can remember way back in medical school, all those rumors and stories of doctors being charged with fraud, or getting a DUI,[5] and then never being able to practice again. The stories frightened me, and I was extra-careful never to put myself at any risk. I would never drive even after a single drink, and I became super honest. I was desperately afraid something I did would lead to a false accusation that might put my career at risk. You're right; we're trained to be almost *too* good. I know I am one of the physicians it sounds like you counsel. When I was first told I needed to document at least 15 specific pieces of medical information to

---

[5]DUI=driving under the influence.

be able to bill for a new patient assessment, I immediately decided 15 was just the minimum, and if I could write more than that, I would be less at risk of failing this billing gauntlet. I guess in that respect it was partly me, and my determination to do things right, that was causing my notes to be excessively long."

"Well, maybe this conversation will help you focus more on the minimum good, quality notes you need to write in the future. I hope it does."

Alexia nodded in agreement. "What you do is fascinating. You must have such an interesting professional life; I'm really quite jealous. I thought all your online work was probably a bit like second-class medicine, just something you do because you travel around the world. Not something you really enjoy and find fulfilling."

"Thanks. That's a very interesting comment. Having been working online in one form or another for several years now, I just see it as another approach to a rewarding professional career. One of the really good things I learned early on, when I first got into telemedicine, is that I actually had more time with my patients because I could write my notes while I was seeing them. That saves time and is much easier on video than it is in person, because it doesn't interrupt your eye contact with the patient. So I ended up spending more time with them overall, which I loved. I realized I also saved 3 or 4 minutes per consultation because there was no clinic-rooming process; I just logged on and started talking to them. It's made me think about how rigid and conservative traditional medical practice is, and how destructive it is to doctors and inconvenient for patients. Our consulting really involves working with physicians and health systems and giving them permission to change. Why do most doctors work business hours when, in fact, patients want to be seen outside business hours? Why can't we be more flexible and in control of our work and our hours? Why do patients have to come to us in a brick-and-mortar world when it's entirely possible for us to go to them using technology, or for us to work in a hybrid manner, both in person and online? When we wish to consult with our colleagues, which is what I do a great deal nowadays, why do we have to travel when we both have access to sophisticated multimedia systems? If we want to educate ourselves about something, why do we go to formal lectures, which are seldom very interactive, when we can use 'just in time' learning online on any topic almost any time? Think of the demise of encyclopedias and the rise of YouTube if you want evidence supporting this educational change. Of course, none of this stops any of us from working in person with our patients in the traditional way. I expect that I will continue with my current work style for the next 5 years or so, but at some stage we'll have to settle down somewhere when the children are old enough for high school. At that point I can see myself changing my work style again. Maybe I'll become a more traditional clinic physician, although I doubt it, because I love the flexibility of my current work."

Just then, the restaurant server came by with dessert, and the topic of conversation moved on to food and children. Alexia signaled to Christina that she wanted to go with her to the restroom. The two friends negotiated the crowds around the bar and made for the women's restroom, where Alexia knew they would be able to talk in private.

"Christina, it's so fascinating listening to you talk about your life," Alexia began. "Is it really as good as you describe? It's hard to believe you are both personally and professionally satisfied. Is that really the case?"

"It really is. I know it's hard to believe, but I really do think I've worked out the work-life balance equation. I have time for my family and children, and I really enjoy my work. Most importantly, I find my work really meaningful. I feel like I'm making a difference. That's why we all went into medicine in the first place, right? I'm so lucky, but it hasn't been that easy, and it hasn't all been as good as it is now. Why do you ask? And why so privately?"

"I've been trying to put on a good face all evening, and being with you and Roberto is so good because you're both so positive and uplifting, which is lovely. But we've been having a much harder time than we told you. Jose talked about us possibly resigning from our jobs, but that's really only half the story. We're being pushed out by the clinic owners. They're putting more and more demands on us both, and on several other doctors in the clinic, and it's clear we have to either knuckle under and see ridiculous numbers of patients per day, essentially practicing bad medicine to meet their requirements for billing totals, or we have to leave. It's corporate medicine at its worst, all driven by the dollar. We have no time during the day to keep up with our EMR work, and because we're both conscientious and really believe in what we're doing for our patients, we do it after hours to make sure our notes are good."

Alexia's face crumpled, and she started crying. "I can't believe it's come to this. Jose and I are always fighting. We're constantly tired. We never do anything nice together. You know, coming out with you tonight is the first date night we've had in more than 2 months. What do you think we do instead?"

"I don't know," answered Christina. "Are you just tired and watching TV?"

"I wish! If only. No, we spend most of our evenings, after the children are in bed, just playing dueling laptops—both of us sitting and catching up on our medical notes and the wretched inbox. We have to answer all direct patient inquiries within 24 hours, and we have no medical assistant support at work since all those staff were fired a few months ago. Jose is more pragmatic about the situation than I am; he started keeping a schedule of the number of hours of work we both do after our notional clinic day, which is usually at least 10–11 hours itself. I was horrified. We both averaged about 15 hours per week extra at nights and on weekends. So when you add up the 55-hour week at work, and this extra 15 hours, we're each working about 70 hours and only get paid for the 40 when we're actually seeing patients. None of this makes any sense. We're trying to work well in the way that we were trained, but it's just impossible. I've done all sorts of reading about our situation, but the cognitive dissonance we're facing, with our belief in good medical practices being contradicted by the need for commercial practices, is just too much."

Alexia started crying again. Tears flowed down her face, smudging her freshly reapplied makeup. Christina put her arms around her and gave her a loving hug while Alexia let off steam and openly expressed her distress. Gradually Alexia calmed down and broke away from Christina, wiping her tear-soaked face with tissues.

"So you see, we have to change. We can't go on working like this, being controlled at work and constantly facing a sea of increasing work and demands. So much of our time is taken up with silly busy work that could be done by others, but the system doesn't understand that and expects us physicians to do all the constantly increasing administrative work. It's all very well to be 'patient focused,' but the way we work, with patients messaging us through the EMR all the time, it just leads to more work for which we aren't compensated. The health system is proud to boast that all its patients have immediate physician access with a 24-hour response time, but we don't get paid to fulfill those mandates. Jose and I are both completely burned out. We've been seeing a therapist to keep our marriage together. We're just not ourselves. It's all too tragic, and I'm so afraid we're not going to make it and stay together. What can we do? How can we change? Please help us."

"I am so sorry," Christina said. "I do know somewhat how you feel. I remember being overwhelmed by the EMR and all those dreadful prior authorizations for drugs that used to take so long. They were just a way for the drug companies to stop us from prescribing anything expensive or unusual, a way to take out all the art in medicine and make us perform as though we follow the same recipe every time. But patients can't be treated that way."

"It's so good to hear that you've managed to get away from all this, from this approach to medicine that feels as though we're tied to a wagon wheel. So many little annoyances and frustrations. Tonight has been interesting. I'm sorry to end up crying like this; I must look like the stereotypical depressed housewife, pouring out her heart in the restroom." She smiled sadly at Christina. "Maybe this is all to the good. I think Jose and I needed a wakeup call, and seeing how we are such a contrast to you guys is just amazing for me. I can't believe how brave you've been to make your career so different from mine. And you've even managed to continue practicing medicine while you've done it, and in such a meaningful way! Three of my former classmates have moved out of medicine altogether in the past year—one into journalism, one to business, and one who simply retired way too early and is traveling by himself after his wife left and took his children away. Jose and I have actually talked about maybe working part-time to give ourselves more time like that, but I don't really think that's an answer. The wakeup call I've had from tonight is that we have to make some changes. You know, I used to have a really good mentor who helped me make career decisions, and I've never forgotten what he used to say to me. He told me that if you're stuck in a career that you don't want, and you don't change the way you work or leave the position, then you're making an active decision to stay. At the time, it really helped me change my decision about residency, because when I saw that by *not* doing something, I still was making a choice, it gave me the strength to plan changes and make alternative choices. I think Jose and I have been making the choice *not* to change our work and lifestyle for too long, and now we have to do something different." She put on a slight smile and looked to Christina. "Enough of that. I think we need to join our husbands. They will have missed us by now and might be worried about what we're plotting in the restroom."

Christina grinned at her friend conspiratorially as they walked out of the restroom and into the noisy restaurant. "Nothing much, really," she teased. "Just aiming to send you and Jose off on a new life together."

Commentary

Four issues of importance arise in this scenario, which contrasts the very different lifestyles of the two couples. The first is the use of information technologies and telemedicine to help physicians work differently and less stressfully. This was discussed in Chapter 4 within a single-clinic setting, whereas in this scenario, Christina runs an international health consulting practice by telemedicine, combining some individual work with a strong emphasis on data analysis to help health systems change strategically. Christina mentioned patient complaints and staff incident reports as being essential to review; when such reports are at a high level, they likely indicate systemic problems within a health care organization and may act as a proxy for burnout in providers. It is possible her consulting company was working closely with the Vanderbilt Center for Patient and Professional Advocacy (ww2.mc.vanderbilt.edu/cppa), whose Patient Advocacy Reporting System and Co-Worker Observation Reporting Systems are evidence-based tools and processes that promote professional accountability and self/group regulation through identifying and intervening with physicians at increased risk for malpractice claims and adverse surgical outcomes. These two quality systems are now in place in about 150 hospital and academic systems in the United States and provide very useful benchmarking data for all involved. A number of other quality systems are in place nationally, such as the Press Ganey (www.pressganey.com) alignment and engagement surveys; thus it is not always necessary to run formal burnout surveys because these other tools may be used as proxies, making the job of consultants like Christina much more straightforward.

The second issue is that of alternative careers from traditional medical practice. Many of these are described in Chapter 10, but Christina's practice is one rarely seen at present. Her career trajectory will likely become more common in future, as technology becomes increasingly less of a barrier and as the constant air travel required in many international companies becomes seen not only as financially expensive and tiring but also as costly from a carbon perspective.

The other two issues here have not been discussed previously. First is climate change and how physicians can contribute to reducing our carbon emissions, thereby improving their own and everyone's well-being. The second is the importance of meaning, and a meaningful life, to physicians and how to overcome the cognitive dissonance many of us face daily and focus on the meaning of our work and careers in a positive, impactful way.

Many physicians and other health providers are becoming increasingly interested in how they can change their work and lifestyle habits in order to reduce the long-term impact of climate change. What are the basic relevant facts, and what changes can individuals and health systems make that will have an impact?

The United States as a whole is a major producer of total carbon dioxide emissions, and the health care sector is responsible for 9.8% of this total (Eckelman and Sherman 2016), which is proportionately less than other industries, and health care consumes 18% of our gross domestic product. Eckelman and Sherman (2016) noted that in the health care industry,

> health damages from these pollutants are estimated at 470,000 DALYs[6] lost from pollution-related disease, or 405,000 DALYs when adjusted for recent shifts in power generation sector emissions. These indirect health burdens are commensurate with the 44,000–98,000 people who die in hospitals each year in the U.S. as a result of preventable medical errors, but are currently not attributed to our health system. Concerted efforts to improve environmental performance of health care could reduce expenditures directly through waste reduction and energy savings, and indirectly through reducing pollution burden on public health, and ought to be included in efforts to improve health care quality and safety.

These numbers should be impossible to ignore. The U.S. health care footprint by itself is larger than the entire footprint from many countries around the world, including the United Kingdom, Brazil, Mexico, and Saudi Arabia. We have to change and reduce our overall carbon footprint at home and at work.

What, then, can individuals do to reduce this communal damage from the impact of climate change? First, we should all measure our carbon footprint (www.conservation.org/act/carboncalculator/calculate-your-carbon-footprint.aspx). Despite thinking that I am fairly energy efficient, I found out that I am not; I produce about 21 tons of carbon per year, approximately the U.S. average, compared with the world average of 7 tons and those of Europe (8 tons) and China and India (4 tons each). The website gives you a series of useful tips to effectively reduce your carbon footprint, which in my case means trying to fly less. For those who wish to examine how their lifestyle and personal choices can reduce their contribution to climate change, Wynes and Nicholas (2017) described concrete choices we can all make, from upgrading lightbulbs (low impact), through recycling and buying a hybrid car (medium impact), to eating a plant-based diet, living car free, avoiding one transatlantic flight, and having one fewer child (all high impact).

What sort of interventions should Christina be recommending to her health system clients to reduce the carbon footprint of health care? We

---

[6]DALYs=disability adjusted life years.

know that the four large carbon-producing areas in the health industry are hospital care, physician and clinical services, prescription drugs, and physical structures and equipment. Activities such as turning off the lights, recycling, and avoiding single-use disposable waste items, which we tend to embrace already, actually save very little carbon overall. So Christina could be advising the following:

1. *Hospital care:* Change volatile anesthetics to sevoflurane to dramatically reduce carbon dioxide emissions by a factor of 20 (Alexander et al. 2018). Reduce food waste and serve less beef and pork.
2. *Clinical services:* Use telemedicine (Holmner et al. 2014; Yellowlees and Shore 2018), mobile devices, and information technologies as much as possible and do not waste or use excess equipment. Avoid unnecessary flying for conferences and meetings.
3. *Prescription drugs:* All drug companies are not the same. Deal with companies that are serious about reducing their carbon impact and are hitting their Paris Accord agreements (Belkhir and Elmeligi 2019). Many are not. Also avoid polypharmacy; give small prescriptions where indicated and take patients off unnecessary medication. Think about social prescribing (Bickerdike et al. 2017) if possible, especially for patients with behaviorally related disorders.
4. *Physical structures and equipment:* Build Leadership in Energy and Environmental Design (LEED)-certified buildings that have good environmental quality and are designed and operated to be centered on people and health requirements (Oaks 2018).

Finally, Christina could quote the University of California (UC)'s Carbon Neutrality Initiative to her customers and suggest that they follow this policy objective. UC, which includes five major medical centers, has long been a leader in sustainability and has now pledged to become carbon neutral by 2025, expecting to become the first major university to accomplish this achievement (Office of the President 2019).

In the discussions in the scenario, the meaningfulness of a medical career was accentuated in the contrast between the work and home lives of the two couples. It was evident that Christina and Roberto were fulfilled by their work and their approach to work, whereas Alexia and Jose were not, suffering from longstanding cognitive dissonance as to the meaning of their work and careers and from burnout.

Why is meaning so important to most of us? What exactly is it, and how can it be improved if it is lacking or missing? These are core questions for the great majority of health care providers, especially physicians, who entered medical school to join a helping profession and to have relationships with and assist patients. Few physicians go to medical school primarily because they want to be rich, and although most appreciate and value the salaries that they earn, they are usually not as valuable to them as the community respect that they gain. Those graduate students who primarily measure their success in life in dollar terms do not tend to go to medical school, preferring business administration or legal routes where they may ultimately earn significantly more than an equivalent doctor.

So what is meaning as it relates to work? How do we define a meaningful job or career? Why is meaning so important for physicians? Dictionaries typically describe *meaning* as being the end, purpose, or significance of something, while *meaningful* is something that is sincere, deep, serious, and important. Not surprisingly, meaning in medicine has been studied by several groups, especially in the setting of burnout and, as described in Chapter 1, in relation to professionalism. This is also a popular topic in many management books and MBA courses and is comprehensively covered by Shell (2014), who focused on whether a work role is really a career, a job, or a calling. He described various definitions of success, ranging from what he called "outer" definitions, such as recognition, achievement, pay, and authority, to "inner" definitions of prosperity such as fulfillment, respect, and happiness. His book will resonate with many physicians who may have desired the inner definitions from their future careers when they entered medical school but have moved over the course of those careers more in the direction of the outer definitions, creating some internal cognitive dissonance or dissatisfaction and possibly symptoms of burnout. Shell also noted that basing a personal definition of success and meaning on "outer" factors such as money and influence is not a recipe for long-term or sustainable happiness and concluded that finding meaningful work consists of the intersection of three core factors. These are:

1. *Work that others will reward you for doing.* This includes many "outer" components such as promotions and status, compensation to meet lifestyle needs, and opportunities for growth.
2. *Work that ignites you emotionally.* This component attracts most physicians and can also be achieved with volunteer work and other after-hours pursuits.
3. *Work that uses your talents and strengths in the service of larger goals.*

If physicians use these factors as guides for finding meaningful positions, and health care as an industry is replete with positions that allow all three core factors to be met, how should individual physicians attempt to measure their own definition of success and fulfillment? Shell defined seven categories that are especially relevant to physicians seeking meaning in their work. In possible order of importance to the typical career of a physician, they are:

1. Personal growth and development—leave your comfort zone and learn new skills to progress.
2. Community care—help others in need and serve a cause bigger than yourself.
3. Talent-based excellence—aspire to become a subject matter expert.
4. Independence—work autonomously and control your own future.
5. Religious or spiritual features—practice your beliefs, faith, or values consistently in service of the greater good.
6. Family involvement and support—provide your loved ones with the means for a better future.
7. Self-expression—pursue ideas, research, teaching, or invention.

In an earlier fascinating qualitative study of physicians, Horowitz et al. (2003) collected 83 stories from internists about what gave them meaning in their professional work. The authors developed three major themes, which they described as follows:

> In the first theme, doctors changed their perspectives about themselves, their roles, human nature, illness, and patient care after being part of a profound event or emotional experience with a patient or sharing or reflecting on their own life experiences. The second theme is about connecting with patients in moments of intimacy. These moments occurred in the course of relationships lasting anywhere from hours to decades, and in settings ranging from mundane to profound. The third and most common theme in the doctors' stories was making a difference in someone else's life. These were success stories, but not of brilliant diagnoses or adroit technical interventions. Most of these stories took place in the context of chronic, incurable conditions, or end-of-life care. In these situations, the doctors themselves were the principal therapeutic agents. They felt awed and deeply rewarded that their mere presence could be healing and comforting to patients. (p. 772)

Perhaps the most important aspect of this study, which bears repetition and may be a useful well-being intervention for others to use, was the authors' conclusion (Horowitz et al. 2003):

> We now have a better and richer understanding of what doctors find meaningful about their work. The internists in our study wrote about miracles and mistakes, sharing their own lives and their patients' lives,

witnessing profound experiences, and receiving acknowledgment for a job well done. Through these events, they were rewarded unexpectedly with a deeper appreciation of what it means to be a human being and a doctor, and of how their caring actions, not just their technical ability, was so important to their patients.

The doctors who participated in our workshops found the process of exchanging stories to be valuable and personally renewing. They experienced a sense of community and reaffirmation. Amid so much discussion of what is wrong with medicine, the workshops seemed to help them remember what is right. With a clearer understanding of what nourishes and sustains them, doctors can be more proactive in advocating for their needs, and, if assured of this, may be more capable of embracing other changes that need to happen. (p. 775)

It is fascinating how this particular study, and the concept of meaning in medicine, is reflected in the process and approach of Balint groups (www.americanbalintsociety.org). A Balint group, developed from the work of Michael Balint in London, is a group of clinicians who meet regularly to present clinical cases in order to improve and to better understand the clinician–patient relationship. Such groups are becoming increasingly popular around the world, partly because of the difficulties that many physicians have working in our current health systems, their cognitive dissonance between how they *wish* to work and how they *have* to work, and the frequent occurrence of symptoms of burnout. Balint groups focus on enhancing the clinician's ability to connect with and care for the patient sustainably, and they may well be one effective solution for improving the lives of physicians by bringing more meaning back to their practice of medicine.

In summary, physicians who recognize similarities between themselves and Alexia and Jose in the scenario should consider reviewing their career directions in light of the concepts of meaning discussed here and perhaps even investigate whether a Balint group exists in their area. Alternatives include thinking about changing practice styles using the many options discussed throughout this book or taking up some rewarding outside interest, such as being involved in the climate change debate and improving the planet.

References

Alexander R, Poznikoff A, Malherbe S: Can J Anesth 65(2):221–222, 2018 29119467

Belkhir L, Elmeligi A: Carbon footprint of the global pharmaceutical industry and relative impact of its major players. J Clean Prod 214:185–194, 2019

Bickerdike L, Booth A, Wilson PM, et al: Social prescribing: less rhetoric and more reality: a systematic review of the evidence. BMJ Open 7(4):e013384, 2017 28389486

Eckelman MJ, Sherman J: Environmental impacts of the U.S. health care system and effects on public health. PLoS One 11(6):e0157014, 2016 27280706

Holmner A, Ebi KL, Lazuardi L, et al: Carbon footprint of telemedicine solutions—unexplored opportunity for reducing carbon emissions in the health sector. PLoS One 9(9):e105040, 2014 25188322

Horowitz CR, Suchman AL, Branch WT Jr, et al: What do doctors find meaningful about their work? Ann Intern Med 138(9):772–775, 2003 12729445

Oaks L: What it takes for healthcare facilities to earn LEED certification. LEED Leadership in Energy and Environmental Design, October 2, 2018. Available at: https://www.laboratoryequipment.com/article/2018/10/what-it-takes-healthcare-facilities-earn-leed-certification. Accessed May 24, 2019.

Office of the President: Carbon Neutrality Initiative (website). University of California, 2019. Available at: https://ucop.edu/carbon-neutrality-initiative/index.html. Accessed May 24, 2019.

Shell RG: Springboard: Launching Your Personal Search for Success. New York, Portfolio, 2014

Wynes S, Nicholas K: The climate mitigation gap: education and government recommendations miss the most effective individual actions. Environ Res Lett 12(7), 2017

Yellowlees P, Shore J: Telepsychiatry and Health Technologies: A Guide for Mental Health Professionals. Washington, DC, American Psychiatric Association Publishing, 2018

Chapter 9

MEDICAL MARRIAGES: CARING FOR EACH OTHER

Scenario

"Please come in, Dr. and Dr. Galvin. Please take the chairs over near the fireplace so we can all be comfortable and talk."

The tall, gray-haired man escorting the two doctors into his office was dressed very casually in his plaid shirt and well-worn khaki pants. He looked compassionately toward the obviously anxious couple as they took their places, and he sat down opposite them.

Marty Canter watched his new patients explore his room with their eyes, trying to pick up clues as to what sort of person he might be. He was unconcerned. His room was comfortable but simply furnished, with one waist-high plant by the single large window and the usual framed degrees validating his profession scattered across the walls. He, and it, had survived the inquisitive looks of many couples over the years without giving too much away. He had an old desk set in the corner of the room; his laptop sat atop it. Heavy velvet curtains hung beside the window, ready to block out the excess summer sun that frequently flooded the room. The main focus was the seating area, the three deep lounge chairs placed around a large fireplace that, although used only occasionally in winter, dominated the room. One wall included a collection of photographs of places across the country where Marty had worked during his long career as a family therapist—no family photos, just buildings. Sometimes his patients asked about the photos, especially the one showing a large, rather forbidding structure that, before it had been demolished, was the psychiatric hospital where he had done his internship many years ago. His first impression of this powerful-looking couple, who seemed very disconnected from each other, was that their focus and interest would be more on themselves, and less on him.

Marty remembered the referral he'd received from his friend of many years, Dr. Jordan Vine, a psychiatrist he had first met during his internship through their mutual love of baseball. Now, they frequently referred patients to each other and often combined their psychiatric and therapy skills, working together to better help their patients. In this instance, he had been at Jordan's home for dinner 2 weeks earlier, and toward the end of the evening Jordan had taken him aside to ask him to see the Galvins, a well-known physician power couple in the city who frequently graced the social pages. Jordan told him that he had been treating Cathy Galvin, a vascular surgeon, for severe depression and that, although she was no longer actively suicidal, during her therapy it had become obvious to him that the couple had some major relationship problems. Jordan had seen Cathy's husband, Brett, a family physician and chair of the local medical society, a couple of times in sessions with Cathy and had discussed marital therapy with them. They had both acknowledged longstanding relationship difficulties and agreed therapy was worth trying, hence his referral to Marty Canter. As they went back to the dinner party group, Jordan added that he was not at all sure that their marriage was salvageable; he wished he could engage Brett in treatment also but the suggestion had been met with a blank refusal and an annoyed, dismissive response that he did not need to see a psychiatrist.

Marty sank into his burgundy leather chair, making himself comfortable, pen and pad in hand for his notes. Cathy Galvin opened the conversation.

"Thank you for seeing us. We understand you're a friend and colleague of Dr. Vine, who speaks highly of you. We're both a bit concerned, though, because you're not a psychiatrist or a psychologist, who mostly have Ph.Ds. We just want to be sure that you understand the special needs that doctors have and the difficult lifestyle and pressures that affect us. Just as patients often ask me how many patients I've operated on for their own problem, I would like to know if you have seen many doctors for therapy?"

Many inexperienced therapists would have been threatened by Cathy's direct and somewhat intimidating approach. Marty just smiled inwardly. He had heard this style of attack many times previously and understood that what could be perceived as arrogance actually often arose from anxiety and Cathy's underlying fear that he would be unable to help them. She had to check him out to reassure herself.

Marty looked carefully at the Galvins. They were both in their early fifties. Cathy had a striking face, long and thin, with dark rings under her large brown eyes that were partially covered by makeup. She had unusually smooth facial skin, possibly from a successful recent facelift, he suspected. Her long, black hair was tied back in a tight ponytail, and she wore a dark, conservative business suit, black pumps, and a single-strand gold necklace. She appeared to be a powerful woman who could have come from any high-level professional occupation, law, engineering, business, or medicine. She sat apart from Brett, her knees and elbows pointing away from him, her body language building an unseen wall. Very intense.

Brett, on the other hand, struck Marty as being much less commanding than his wife. He looked tired and rather beaten down, a bit like a faithful spaniel who has lost his way but is trying to keep up with his master. He seemed less certain of himself and made little eye contact. He looked his age, with blotchy skin and his share of wrinkles, but his long, carefully styled white hair suggested that a hair dryer might be in regular use. Like his wife, he wore a perfectly tailored suit and polished black leather shoes, all finished off with a Rolex watch that gleamed on his left wrist.

They were an interesting couple. He sensed that they both would rather be anywhere but in his office today. Marty wondered about the details of their journey together and whether they could be helped. He decided to reassure Cathy first and then start exploring why they were consulting him.

"I understand your concern, Cathy, because you're right, it is important to understand the culture of medicine, the realities of the world you live in and the pressures on you both as a result. Because I am a marital therapist who regularly sees physicians, I have a good understanding of the other extra pressures that occur within any marriage of two physicians, especially the juggling of competing careers and schedules and how these may intrude on family and home life. I understand that you both work in very different areas of medicine, surgery and family medicine, and I would guess that those issues have been important to you both over the years. Is that the case?"

"They certainly have been," said Brett, "but I think we've managed to overcome a lot of those difficulties. Certainly, my career in family medicine has helped because I've been able to be more flexible than Cathy. The surgical training, especially for a female, is simply murderous. We decided not to have children, for instance, until Cathy had finished her residency because of her long, unpredictable hours and because the hospital where she was training didn't have good childcare facilities. It would have been almost impossible for us to manage children at that time of our careers with our shift work."

"I've heard a lot of doctors complain about the difficulties of bringing up children with the required schedules," said Marty sympathetically. "How many children do you have, and how old are they?"

"Two. James is 12, and Sashi is 10," said Cathy. "We were actually very fortunate to have them because I was a relatively mature mother at the time, after finishing my fellowship in vascular surgery. Fortunately, they're both fit and well, although we did have a very hard time with James, who was mistakenly diagnosed with microcephaly—a very small skull—when I was pregnant. I think that was the first time we really had major problems in our marriage. I'll never forget being alone while having the ultrasound that led to the mistaken diagnosis. I had to discuss the possibility of a termination without Brett there because he was stuck in clinic with an acutely ill patient he couldn't leave. I think I blamed him for that for months, even after James had been born completely healthy. I was just so used to attending all my OBGYN[1] appointments by myself. Suddenly I realized most of the other prospective mothers had their partners with them for at least some of the visits. I know it's the life we signed up for, but it's been tough at times. It may sound odd, but sometimes we're lonely because we're both doctors and have commitments that pull us apart. We have so often had to be that way—just one parent available for our children at a schoolteachers night, sports day, or the first day of school. We've become excellent schedule jugglers, but only so that one of us can get to these events. Sadly, for me and for the children, Brett usually has been the parent present. He's been really good about that, but it hit home to me when one of the parents in

---

[1]OBGYN=obstetrics and gynecology.

James's class asked Brett if he was a single parent. I wish I could have been there for the children more."

Cathy sat back, suddenly overcome with emotion. She felt like crying but forced herself to maintain control and not show her reactions too openly. This was something she had learned over many years in surgery: to keep herself emotionally distant from the many awful traumas she experienced so she could better support and advise her patients. She was surprised at herself for being so open with this stranger about one of her greatest disappointments in life—being more absent than she would have liked in the lives of her children. It felt odd.

"That sounds rotten, Cathy. I appreciate how difficult that must have been for you," Marty responded. "However, I imagine that this must have been only one of a number of difficulties you've both had, or you wouldn't be here. Could one of you tell me a bit more, so I have a fuller picture? And please remember that, as a marital therapist, I won't be taking sides in any of this. It's my job to work with you both to try to resolve any problems that you wish to discuss. Of course, some issues between you may arise that you don't want to include in our discussions, and I will certainly respect those boundaries."

Brett decided it was time to give his perspective. Lifting his head and taking a deep breath, he jumped into the conversation.

"Cathy and I have been married since medical school. We met early in our first year and rapidly became inseparable. In my view, Cathy is more intelligent and ambitious, and I think if you can get her to be honest, she will agree on that. She always wanted to be a surgeon. Even in medical school, she was determined to be the star student. She was on the dean's honors list and has always worked incredibly hard, so it was no surprise when she got into a prestigious surgical training program. Fortunately, I was able to follow her and obtained a residency in family medicine on a partners program. In some respects, I've always felt like the person who has to pick up the pieces behind Cathy as she becomes more and more highly trained and successful. We had large debts from medical school, about $400,000 between us, and they really overshadowed our first 5 years after residency when we were both working extralong hours to pay them off. At the same time, we were trying to start a family, which took several years. I've always thought we were just too stressed for conception to be successful quickly."

"That, combined with my night work schedule, meant we were only together a few nights a week, and I was always exhausted," said Cathy. "So don't just blame stress. If you remember, we weren't actually having sex that often either, then or since, so it's not surprising it took a while for me to become pregnant."

"Please, Cathy. I don't think we need to get into that level of detail here!" said Brett, rapidly and in an irritated voice. "It's the problems we've been having over the past 5 years that are really why we're here, as we both discussed. Or do you want to cover different areas? I, for one, do not want to go back over ancient history. It cannot be relevant now."

Brett looked angry and suddenly more assertive, emerging from his initially dependent, passive role and glaring at his wife before turning away from her to look directly at Marty. Surprised at how quickly the temperature between the couple had increased, Marty decided to intervene. He sensed an escalating dispute occurring as Cathy drew farther away from Brett and showed her own anger in her body language.

"I'm sure we'll have time at some stage to go over numerous issues. Sexual problems certainly are common in most relationships that are having difficulties and can be either a symptom or a cause. Let's go back to why you both think you're here. Perhaps it would be best if you could individually talk about that directly to each other, letting me be the observer. That way, we can clear the air and identify more precisely what you both feel and think and where we should start working. Who would like to go first?"

"Okay," said Cathy. "I've already been branded as the ambitious workaholic in our marriage, so I'll take the first shot at this." She turned to Brett, moving her whole body around, crossed her legs in a business-like way, and looked him directly in the eyes. "Brett, one thing that frustrates me is that you're always trying to please everyone, and putting me last, because you're so used to me being able to cope. You're a great family doctor; you go out of your way to help all of your patients. Nothing is too much for you. You are the same with our children; you seem to love the fact that their teachers automatically go to you first for any parenting questions. And you're proud of being what others think of as a 'hero' because you cover for me so much of the time and are the perfect dad. So they all admire you and think I'm not being a good mom. That's how the public sees you."

She paused, seemingly to take a short break, but Marty wondered if her pause was also for effect. When she continued, she spoke carefully and in a way that seemed almost rehearsed. If not rehearsed, then it certainly was well thought through and calculated.

"Brett, your private face is different from your public persona. You're not nearly as good at coping as others think. I see all the hours of work you do at home to make sure your medical records are up to date.

I know how difficult it's been for you to adapt to the EMR,[2] but how you won't admit it and get extra help or coaching. Instead, you spend half your weekends trapped on the EMR, communicating with your patients by messaging. *Of course* they all think you're wonderful if you respond to them at 10 P.M. on a Sunday. I see you looking exhausted, and lately I've noticed you're drinking too much, almost always polishing off a bottle of wine every evening. You never used to do that. I've talked to you about your drinking many times, and you won't acknowledge it or even go and see a colleague to be checked out. Why, you don't even have a family physician yourself, although you tell all your patients to make sure they always have regular checkups with you! We both know you have some erectile dysfunction, perhaps caused by your drinking, and as a result you avoid intimacy with me. Maybe your charting at home is just a convenient excuse to avoid spending time with me. So, my main point is that I want you to start looking after yourself better. And I want to be looked after as well, and not used as a reason for you to look good to others. I'm sick of you working on the EMR at home and wish you could finish your work *at work*, so you can be a dad and a husband at home. I know I'm not perfect, and I'm sure you'll talk about that, but I really do want us to succeed and stay together. It's as though we've become more like roommates than a couple, and that has to change. That is what I want from coming here, to try to get us back on track. That's why Dr. Vine sent us here."

"I know why we're here, Cathy. You don't need to remind me," Brett replied tersely. "You seem to have Dr. Vine on a pedestal. We have to do exactly what he suggests, because he can't be wrong. I know you think he's perfect in comparison with me. I can't believe you've needed all those appointments with him to just talk about yourself. I see how you always dress up to go and see him. Do you know that sometimes hearing you describe him is like listening to an adolescent girl with a crush? All I can say is that I know you think I'm overly suspicious of you, but that's hardly surprising, considering you have *admitted* to having at least one affair in the past. I've asked you a dozen times to see a different psychiatrist, and you always refuse on the grounds that he saved your life when you were seriously suicidal. I think you have a thing for him, and he comes between us. I don't want to feel like I'm in second place."

"You're being unfair, Brett. I thought we'd worked through that one time I messed up. It didn't mean anything, and you know it. I was drunk,

---

[2]EMR=electronic medical record.

and it was one night. I think you've beaten me up enough on that one. It was 5 years ago! This is complete nonsense. How often do I have to tell you? Dr. Vine is my psychiatrist, and that's all. I know you're worried that I will repeat the past. Can't you ever get over that one mistake of mine? You told me you were over it, and now you throw it at me again. I was desperate at the time and have promised it would never happen again. I have felt awful and so guilty about what I did that night. But here you are, within a few minutes of meeting a therapist who's meant to help us, bringing up old ground once again. You know exactly what happened, and I promise all that is in the past. We need to concentrate on now. And I am going to continue seeing Dr. Vine as my doctor because he has helped me so much." Cathy angrily turned away from Brett, clearly disconsolate and distressed. She grabbed a tissue from her bag to wipe away some newly forming tears. "Why don't you do what Marty suggests and summarize what we've discussed and why you think we're here. Please let go of that ancient history. As far as I'm concerned, it was dead and buried many years ago."

Marty intervened. It was obvious Cathy and Brett were furious with each other. He decided to look for a more neutral area in which to engage, to try to reduce the growing strain between them, but he felt the need to reassure Brett first.

"Brett, Cathy seems clear about her view of Dr. Vine, and I can reassure you that he, and his wife, Pat, have been among my closest friends for 30 years. If anything inappropriate had happened between Cathy and Dr. Vine, he would most certainly not have referred you both to me. Doctors who have affairs with patients get reported to the medical board. We both know that boundary violations in the doctor–patient relationship are unforgivable."

"Thank you, Marty. I appreciate you saying that," said Cathy. "Unfortunately, Brett imagines all too often that I'm having affairs whenever I'm away or on call. He makes regular accusations about several colleagues, as well as Dr. Vine. It's true, I did have that one stupid night that I will always regret. I'm not proud of that, and Brett knows it. He just can't seem to forgive me and move on. He's like a dog with a bone where that one incident is concerned and constantly brings it up, blaming me for everything wrong between us. I can't stand this continuing and have been trying really hard to change. That's why I started seeing Dr. Vine more than 5 years ago, because we kept fighting over the famous one night!"

"Forgive me, but you must have other reasons for seeing Dr. Vine," Marty replied. "Have you been seeing him regularly for the past 5 years?

What sort of therapy or medication management has he used with you? He didn't fill me in on your background so as not to bias me in any way. As a marital therapist, it's best that I start my work with an open mind, not influenced by what might be inaccurate perceptions of one member of the couple. Perhaps you could tell me why you've been seeing him, and then we will move back to Brett and hear why he thinks you're both here. Is that okay?"

"Certainly," said Cathy. "From my perspective, my seeing Dr. Vine is a major part of why we're here. I can honestly say that he has saved my life; had I not been seeing him for treatment, I think I would have eventually killed myself. I've been in such dark places. Brett knows all of this story, and I've tried to be as honest with him as possible. He's come to see Dr. Vine with me on several occasions and knows he's welcome to come anytime he wants. I think his jealousy of me is driven by his alcohol abuse, but he refuses to accept that.

"It took me about a year to finally build up the courage to reach out to Dr. Vine, and I only went because a surgical colleague approached me and took me out for coffee. This was one of the senior surgeons in my department, and he told me that he and several of his colleagues had become worried about me and thought I was burned out. He knew something was wrong with me. He was very empathic and respectful; he didn't try to make me talk at length, but he did a great job of pointing out how different I'd become from the colleague he had known previously. He said that it was obvious I'd lost weight, and I was looking tired, was more irritable than usual, and seemed to be less interested in my work. He said some of the operating room nurses had also approached him about me because I'd become so touchy and quick-tempered with them, and they thought I might be depressed. Anyway, I ended up in tears in front of him in the coffee shop. It was so embarrassing. But I knew I had to do something. I talked to Brett about breaking down and thinking I should see someone professionally, and he was very supportive, of course. The perfect husband. He always is, as long as he looks good and is seen as helpful. Except in this case he didn't know half of what I was feeling at the time, although he does now."

Brett interrupted, speaking in a more conciliatory manner. "What Cathy says is true. She was amazing at hiding her feelings and the level of her depression at the time. I really had no idea. She'd always been so self-confident and capable; her seeing herself as weak and starting to think about suicide as the solution to her problems was something I would never have imagined. Thank goodness we had James and Sashi— I think Cathy actually might have killed herself if we didn't."

"Brett's right. Without James and Sashi, I would likely have suicided. That's how bad it had become. I felt awful all the time. I actually had it all planned out by the time I went to see Dr. Vine. I remember thinking that all I had to do was fool him, as I had everyone else, including Brett. Then I'd be free to just end it all, in the knowledge that Brett would look after the children fine. I didn't think much of psychiatrists, so I thought fooling him would be easy. But that's not what happened."

They continued discussing their longstanding mutual problems for some time. As the session concluded, Marty summarized the problem areas he had identified and set them some homework discussions to have before the next session. Three months and nine sessions later, Marty spoke to Cathy and Brett.

"Congratulations on reaching your tenth session of therapy. I have to say that, at the beginning, I wasn't sure you would get this far. But you've been very honest with each other and have both made real efforts to change. I think this would be a good time to review what's happened and how you're feeling about each other, as well as to look forward and talk about your future some more. Are you okay with that?"

As usual, Cathy spoke first, turning toward Brett to address him directly, as they had both learned to do during the sessions. "Well, I think the first hurdle for you, Brett, was learning to trust me again. Marty's idea for you to visit Dr. Vine with me and to specifically ask Dr. Vine about your fears of me having a relationship with him, as well as any other questions you had, was really helpful. His explanation of how he used the doctor–patient relationship as part of therapy, to help patients understand other relationships and parallels in their lives, seemed to reassure you. But the thing that made the greatest difference was when he told you how serious I had been about suicide, something I had never told you because I was so ashamed of myself. It's now out in the open that I'd gone so far as to steal a supply of the anesthetic propofol and some drip sets from work and book a room for myself at a motel 100 miles from home on my next birthday. I'd planned to put the drip up on myself and open the line so that I gradually went to sleep. I'd planned a painless death, rather like the one our vet gave Mitzi when he euthanized her the year before. The first time I saw Dr. Vine, I was in the middle of writing letters to Sashi and James and struggling with the sort of advice I could give them going forward because they were so young and would not likely remember me well. I knew I could kill myself in peace once that was done. At work, I was concentrating on finishing a number of outstanding projects so that I could go with my life nicely tied up— everything completed, neat and clean, just like a good operation."

Cathy paused and gathered her thoughts. "My first appointment with Dr. Vine was about 6 weeks before the date of my planned suicide. No one knew my plans, certainly not you. I think it's been helpful in the past few weeks for you to understand how I felt. I've finally been able to be completely honest with you about this. In the past I just glossed over my suicide plans, and you didn't like to ask, but now it's out in the open, and that's been freeing for me. I've always wondered what your reaction would be if you discovered the extent of my plans. I expected you to be angry and revolted that I could be so selfish, that you would blame and discard me. But you haven't been like that, and I really thank you for not rejecting me now that you know my deepest secret. You've been very forgiving and loving and have really surprised me, so I'm seeing you now in a different light. I think we're better with each other. I'm also glad you've slowed down so much on the wine. I'm glad it's more a special occasion thing instead of an every-night thing. Thank you."

Brett smiled an acknowledgment. Marty thought he seemed younger and more relaxed, less on edge and passively angry. In that vein, Brett looked directly at Cathy and responded to her gratitude.

"I'm so pleased, Cathy. Thank you for telling me. Reducing my drinking went hand in hand with us stopping all the fighting and starting to just talk openly with each other. I was blown away by what you told me about your suicide plans. I had no idea you were so serious. Even after you told me that you'd been suicidal, I was always afraid to ask about your suicide plans and what you intended. There's so much stigma about that, and I already knew you were ashamed to be seeing a psychiatrist. I thought talking about suicide and your other deeply held fears might just make you worse, so I tried to ignore all that and assumed Dr. Vine would deal with it. I guess at one level I was right. I remember you coming home furious from your first appointment with him when he'd explained that he would be treating you like any other intelligent patient and would not be taking any shortcuts just because you were a physician. You'd been able to play the physician card very successfully with everyone else, but not with him. He ended up asking in detail about your depression and suicidal ideas and plans in a way that no one else had ever contemplated talking to you about, and you told him. I know part of you wanted to live. He connected with that part of you and treated your depression with medication and therapy. Now that I know how seriously ill you were, and how he really did save your life, I am much more grateful to him. I think up until recently I didn't understand the depth of your illness and why you'd been seeing him for so long. I was truly jealous of your relationship with him, and I *was* afraid you might have an affair with him at some point. I see now that I had no reason for such ideas. I just didn't know how miserable you were." He smiled lovingly at Cathy before going on. "It's been lovely these past few weeks. I feel like we're talking together again the way we did in medical school, like we can both trust each other again."

"It's good to hear you both being so positive about each other," said Marty, keen to acknowledge the increased trust that both Cathy and Brett were showing. "What other achievements do you think you've made in the past 3 months? Can you summarize any other changes?"

Unusually, this time Brett spoke up first. "I think the session we had about a month ago, when we focused on what we actually do at home, and why, was especially helpful. I've started to make a few changes in my life as a result, and I think Cathy has too. Writing a diary about the times we're at home and what we do during those times was so helpful. Having us both do it so we could compare was a bit frightening, but it really made it clear that we had to decide to change, or not to change, which is what we'd been doing previously. We both decided to change."

Cathy joined in. "We have markedly reduced the amount of EMR work we do in the evening. You pointed out that this was one way we might be hiding from each other, and I think you were right. For me, it was easier because I have fewer clinic patients to see, which is where the notes are a killer, but now I'm making an effort to finish all my notes at work. Before, I left them unfinished, almost like an excuse to have something to do in the evening instead of spending time with Brett after the children were in bed. Brett has made a huge effort, though. He has finally gotten some coaching from the EMR super-users at work to make him more efficient, and he's working with a colleague to reduce the amount of documentation they do per patient, all to reduce his 'pajama time' on the EMR at night. And he really has cut that back, so now he's only doing 3 or 4 hours per week, all of which he is noting and monitoring so he can try to reduce further."

"That's right," said Brett. "I think I was in a rut, where I'd just given up on the EMR and couldn't see a way to save time. And it was an excuse for the evenings, of course. I know it's going to take me a while to manage all my notes without after-hours work, but I think I can succeed. The part I've really changed is in my responses to patients. Now I tell them I'll respond within 24 hours, rather than immediately, so most of my inbox messages are handled at work rather than late at night. One of my patients actually sent me a note congratulating me for not responding immediately on a Sunday afternoon. She said she'd been worrying about me being always available, always tied to a computer.

What an irony! I was trying to provide excellent, fast service, and my patients were worrying I wasn't looking after myself!" Brett laughed. "Anyway, you'll be glad to know that, at your suggestion, Cathy and I are really making some concrete changes in our lifestyle. We've taken up tennis again, like we used to play 15 years ago. We've found a nice mixed-doubles evening tournament that we've joined, and we're playing twice a week. Our first games were last week, and we were both pretty rusty, but we enjoyed the matches and even won a couple of sets. I hope we'll get to play regularly. You were right when you talked about us doing things together that we enjoy and planning some evenings for ourselves. Next week we're going on a date night as soon as we have a babysitter confirmed, and we've sat down with Sashi and James to talk about a family vacation to Cape Cod in a few months. We found a house for rent there that's a block from the beach."

"That all sounds very positive, Cathy and Brett," said Marty. "It sounds like you're communicating so much better. Just keep remembering that almost all your work as a couple should be occurring between sessions. The times we have together are mainly for discussing progress, reviewing, and planning."

"I think we both understand that well, Marty," said Cathy. "But I'd like to bring up one other issue that affects us both and that I'd like to discuss because I think we could make some more changes there."

"Sure, what is it?"

"Well, it's a common problem that affects many doctors. How many events and social activities are we doing both individually and as a couple that we really enjoy, or just doing because we think we should? Especially because they take us away from the children at night and on weekends. Let me give you some examples for both of us. Brett is chair of the local community medical group. That's a very prestigious volunteer position, but it involves several evening meetings each month, usually by himself, and a lot of extra phoning and administrative stuff that comes with the role. I know he enjoys it, and it's a big deal, but it takes up family time. I'm just as bad; I'm on several charity boards and somehow got involved with organizing fundraisers. Although my photo gets in the papers, which is good for my surgical practice, it's still time consuming and keeps me out at night. I'd like to have a series of discussions over the next few weeks about these issues to see if we can start making some changes. After all, with our tennis nights, and doing more things with the children, I don't see how either of us will have time for these sorts of activities. The club where we're playing tennis provides free childcare and a great play yard, which works well for us. We can all go together to the club and usually make it a pizza night together. I would prefer we concentrate on our family and the few really good friends we have than on all the acquaintances we seem to meet through our present activities."

"Good point, Cathy," said Brett. "I must say that I agree with you. I think we've both gotten into a cycle where we've overextended ourselves over the years. I didn't realize how many evenings we were spending on outside events each month. I'm fine with cutting those back and won't miss the charity balls at all!" He laughed.

Cathy smiled. "And equally so, I'm fine with missing the evening meetings to welcome new members of the Medical Society. It's time for another volunteer. I'm so much happier at home these days with you and the kids."

"Okay Marty, it seems like we have at least one new task on our agenda for the upcoming sessions!" said Brett. "It sounds like we both want to focus our time and energies on the people who are important to us. We can't continue to spread ourselves thin across many people and groups, as you have observed in the past. Incidentally, we had a funny conversation with Sashi last night that I think you'll enjoy hearing about. For a 10-year-old, Sashi is old beyond her years, and she constantly impresses us with how worldly she is. She's quite a contrast with James, who's only interested if the conversation involves objects that are round and bounce."

Cathy laughed. "He likes oblong footballs too!"

"Of course," Brett laughed. "Anyway, Sashi approached us in the kitchen after dinner last night, once James had left us to watch sports. She wanted to know if we really had rented the house in Cape Cod, because she wanted to pack—even though it's not planned for another month! We asked why she wanted to pack so soon and why she thought we hadn't really booked it. Sashi told us that she couldn't remember a whole week's vacation with us before and was just excited and wanted to get ready. That really hit us both hard. She was right; Sashi was 2 years old the last time we went on a family vacation for an entire week. Going forward, we agreed to plan annual vacations for at least 2 weeks with the kids. Sashi's face lit up with the biggest smile."

Turning specifically to Marty, Brett went on. "I know we've given you a bit of a hard time on occasions, but we really appreciate what you're doing. We talked a lot about Sashi's reaction last night, and I guess we must be going in the right direction. So thank you."

Commentary

This is the first scenario to focus on medical marriages and some of the many specific stressors faced by doctors who are in relationships with other doctors. These relationships are not always easy, despite the potential advantage of both partners understanding the culture of medicine, which usually brings its own baggage to any relationship involving a physician. In this scenario, Cathy and Brett discussed problems with finding quality time together; career complications; chronic family scheduling difficulties, especially around parenting requirements and childcare; financial burdens that had led to delayed decisions and gratification; the need to show a positive public persona; and the expectations of leadership roles in the community. As a couple, they demonstrated the way many physicians hide behind their work, often using the EMR as an excuse instead of learning to tame it properly and denying emotional and relationship problems. In this scenario, Cathy, the stereotypical female surgeon, unfortunately reported just how inappropriately brutal some training programs can be and still are. Other issues that might be discussed include the effect of student debt burdens, the need for many physicians to receive good financial advice, and how physicians can best approach colleagues in distress. Finally, yet again we see the issue of stigma surrounding psychiatry and the refusal of many physicians like Brett to seek care. His alcohol abuse, denial, and lack of a primary care physician were major barriers to his well-being.

Given that about 40% of physicians marry other physicians or another health professional (American Medical Association Physician Communications Team 2019), what do we know about medical marriages? What are the positive and the negative aspects?

On the positive side, it's not surprising that doctors tend to marry other doctors, if only because of life's timing and the tendency to be seeking a life partner at the same time one is going through medical school or residency. It is at these transitional times in life that social arrangements tend to be made with other student or resident colleagues, as happened with Cathy and Brett. Long hours spent at work with friends in the school or hospital contribute further, as do developing common interests and shared experiences, values, and passions. A recent American Medical Association document described the importance for some physicians of finding someone who shared their perspective on medicine and understood why it is necessary to go to work at Christmas or in the middle of the night but who can also listen and communicate easily about frustrations or difficulties at work (American Medical Association Physician Communications Team 2019).

Medscape, in their "Physician Lifestyle, Happiness, and Burnout Report 2019" (Kane 2019), examined physician relationships via a survey of more than 15,000 physicians in 29 specialties and concluded that most physicians still enjoy medicine and have rich personal lives. They found that three-quarters of physicians reported being happy outside of work, compared with a national poll of all Americans in which only one-third of respondents said they were happy, and that male physicians overall reported much higher self-esteem than females, possibly related to the extra difficulties female doctors experience in obtaining career advancement as well as their tendency to more frequently acknowledge their insecurities, as shown by Cathy in the scenario. Of the physicians who responded to the survey, 85% reported being married or in a committed relationship, with 7% single and 7% divorced. Among those who were married, both males and females, 84% described their marriage as good and 15% described it as fair or poor; 18% reported being married to a physician and 27% to a nonphysician health professional.

On the other side of the coin, however, are the inevitable challenges that physician couples face, like those Cathy and Brett described. Childcare and difficult schedules, especially shifts, are often massive problems for these couples, making it hard to strike a good work-life balance, never mind simply the lack of time spent together. As Mike Drummond (2014), whose nom de plume is the HappyMD, says, "without boundaries, the practice is like an 800-pound gorilla and simply takes over all the available bandwidth." Patients also intrude emotionally, especially when sentinel events, difficult relationships, or poor clinical outcomes are happening that can take most of a physician's emotional energy, leaving little left for partners or family. Also, with high burnout levels in the profession generally, a pair of married doctors is more than likely at some stage to have one partner affected by burnout; depression, such as Cathy experienced; or alcohol use disorder, like Brett. Childcare and parenting roles are often very problematic for professional couples, especially if both are on shift work and working 60–80 hours per week. Residency occurs during a time in the lives of many couples when they also wish to start a family, and some, like Brett and Cathy, choose to delay becoming pregnant as a result. However, this can lead to future concerns as female physicians battle the time clock and eventually begin having children in their late thirties or later. Nannies and childcare do not always work well with shift work, especially on nights and weekends, and in some states childcare services are only legally allowed to take children for a maximum of 45 hours per week, making logistics more complicated. Thus, although physicians may earn good salaries after residency and can afford to pay for childcare (assuming they are also covering their student debt payments), the practicalities can be very challenging.

Although having shared traits and passions can certainly be positive, being too similar, especially when this involves denying emotionally important issues, can be negative and may lead to a tendency not to confront or work through problems. Also, the power balance within a physician–physician marriage can be difficult. Most physicians are used to being powerful and the ultimate team deciders at work and may find this authority hard to relinquish at home.

What, then, should physician couples do to either improve their marriages or prevent them ending in divorce, as is the case for 50% of all marriages in America? Hopefully, not all couples will end up seeing a marital therapist, as in the scenario, and will take action much earlier in their relationships. A number of interesting reference books have been written on the specific topic of medical marriages that are worth reviewing, notably by Myers (1994), Gabbard and Menninger (1988), and Sotile and Sotile (2000). Between them, these books have many good points about how to manage and balance marriages such as described in the scenario. They review the stresses inherent within a medical marriage and how to overcome these, especially the difficulties of managing two potentially all-enveloping, high-powered careers and the inevitable mutual anger and conflict that can arise, hidden or overt, over time. In contrast to this are all the positives that come within a healthy, high-powered relationship and how, with appropriate nurturing and careful communication, such relationships have advantages over many marriages with many very positive aspects, socially and financially, that allow the partners to rise above the inherent competitive elements.

Hans and Kavita Arora, a young and thoughtful physician couple, described several principles that they adapted from advice given to them. These tips would have been very helpful to Cathy and Brett had they upheld them throughout their marriage (Arora and Arora 2018). The principles they suggested are as follows:

1. Prioritize each other in the long term. Although it may not be possible to spend as much time with your medical spouse for a few days, make sure that in the long term you achieve balance by choosing to excel at being good spouses as you rotate through your various roles.

2. Delegate noncrucial tasks both at work and at home, especially using your financial stability to outsource household tasks such as cleaning and laundry.
3. Share hobbies that allow you not only to do something you enjoy but also to spend time with the one you love.
4. Compromise to ensure equality both at work and at home.
5. Share your financial values and goals. Use a financial planner or other advisor and develop a shared vision of your short- and long-term financial picture.
6. Share your professional goals in frank, honest discussions about what success looks like, and revisit these discussions periodically.

These principles are an excellent guideline for any marriage of busy professionals, but what should medical couples do about the negative side of the medical marriage, where lack of time together is a major issue? Drummond (2014) had some useful tips for how to combat the medical practice, which he described as being like a jealous lover that gets in the way of all marriages. He suggested that to carve out more time for a relationship, it is helpful to

1. Create a life calendar as a couple, with specific time carved out as time together.
2. Have date nights at least twice per month, planned at least 3 months in advance, including dinner when not on call, and with all phones turned off.
3. Buy season tickets for events that you both enjoy, and attend them.
4. Create and perform a mindfulness exercise as a boundary ritual between work and home so you do not worry about work while at home.
5. Plan vacations and pay for them in advance so you are more likely to take them rather than find some excuse to cancel at the last moment.

Of course, medical marriages share the same components at their core as all other marriages, and although literally thousands of books and articles describe how to have a successful marriage, Hillin (2014) summarized what she called 13 simple tricks to a long and happy marriage:

1. Be nice.
2. Enjoy each other's company.
3. Say "I love you" as much as possible.
4. Be honest.
5. Limit outside influences, especially from in-laws.

6. Make frequent, small demonstrations and tokens of love.
7. Have some alone time—it makes the heart grow fonder.
8. Be realistic; don't expect 100% all the time. Remember the 80/20 rule and try to give at least 80% of expectations.
9. Cherish each other, and do not take each other for granted.
10. Be your own person; you are separate individuals with your own opinions and tastes.
11. Build a strong foundation of friendship.
12. Know that relationships are a two-way street.
13. No marriage is perfect. You will have and work through disagreements, and that is okay.

Given the high number of physicians who marry other physicians or health care providers, and how we know that a good marriage is protective of physician health and well-being, it seems logical that education about physician marriages and relationships should be part of every core curriculum at medical school and in residency. It is, sadly, rather remarkable that it is not. The absence of this core topic in the medical education system is similar to the frequent absence of education on finances, both personal and practice, and especially on the impact of student debt on early career physicians. In the scenario, Cathy and Brett deliberately delayed having children until they had paid off a combined debt of about $400,000, which is not an unusual amount for a married physician couple. Imagine the pressure, both individually and on a marriage, of being in your early to midthirties, with 12–15 years of training behind you, and carrying debt that is equivalent to the size of a mortgage before you even attempt to buy a home.

What are the financial debt issues facing physicians, and how do they drive career choices? The Association of American Medical Colleges (2018) estimated that 75% of the medical student class of 2018 graduated with educational debt. These students had an average debt of $196,000, with 16% having a debt level greater than $300,000; 46% planned to enter a loan forgiveness repayment program whereby they would, over a 10-year period including residency, work in publicly nominated positions (usually government, military, or universities) where salaries are typically less. They would make the minimum debt repayments over those 10 years, and at the end of that time, the remainder of their debt would be forgiven. Not surprisingly, these loan-forgiveness repayment programs are popular, but they mean that newly qualified doctors post residency have fewer career choices than they had originally hoped for and may end up taking what they might see as second-choice positions at the beginning of their careers. Even for those who are not on such programs, debt is well known to drive career choices. In recent years, a large number of residency applications have been made to what are often known as "lifestyle specialties" such as dermatology, anesthesiology, ophthalmology, and radiology, where the pay is good and work hours are relatively short, with little time on-call, meaning better work-life balance and the opportunity to repay debt quickly. Perhaps surprisingly, psychiatry, for many years a discipline that was relatively unpopular among medical students applying for residency, is now being added to this list of perceived lifestyle specialties. The numbers of psychiatry residency applications has substantially increased in recent years; in 2018, there were significantly more applicants than available places nationally.

Physicians traditionally have a reputation for being poor personal finance managers. Not surprisingly, this is often related to a history of 15 or more years of relative poverty followed by a sudden transition into a position where they are very well paid. Many lack the skills or understanding to manage this new environment and tend to spend excessive amounts of money on short-term rewards, often incurring more debt and financial leverage, with little long-term planning. As such, physicians' postresidency periods become targets for many marketing approaches designed to separate them from their money. Think of all the schemes involving part ownership of racehorses that physicians take up with alacrity. Equally, many an entrepreneur has found physicians keen to invest in high-risk schemes with little understanding of the potential downside and losses. Such is the natural reaction to suddenly becoming "rich" without the financial tools or knowledge to manage this new situation. To prove this to yourself, search "physician wealth services" on Google and see just how many thousands of financial advisors and wealth "solutions" exist that specifically target physicians.

Medscape has created an annual report of physician wealth and debts, and the 2018 report, with responses from more than 20,000 physicians in 29 specialties, makes fascinating reading (Kane 2018). Physicians are certainly well paid, with an average salary in 2018 for all specialties of $299,000 and specialists, on average, having both a larger salary range than primary care practitioners and earning 48% more. With those salaries, however, only 5% of physicians have a net worth (including all assets) of more than $5 million, while 58% have a net worth of less than $1 million. Not surprisingly, the five highest-earning specialties (plastic surgery, radiology, orthopedics, cardiology, and gastroenterology) correlated with the highest proportion of net worth above $2 million, whereas younger physicians, with more debt, less

built-up savings, and less home equity make up most of the 39% of physicians reporting a net worth below $500,000. Physicians tend to reach
their peak net worth after age 50, by which time most medical school
loans have been paid off. Female physicians earn less, take more leave,
and tend to receive lower-paying positions when they return to the
workforce than male physicians. About 6% of physicians reported that
they outspend their income, but another 50% said they live "at their
means," leaving less opportunity for saving or building wealth; 13% reported that they put no money into tax-deferred savings accounts. Only
half of the respondents had a specific savings goal, such as a projection
of costs and income in retirement. Most have worked with a financial
planner at some stage, although only 40% said they were doing so at the
time of the survey and about half reported at least one failed investment.

What can we conclude from these brief facts? Physicians have the
opportunity to be very financially comfortable in life, despite large education debts, but a surprisingly small proportion reach the level of financial success and independence that their salaries might predict,
especially females. Evidence supports the notion that financial needs
drive career specialty decisions, although given the possible salaries
achievable across the board, if physicians were better financially educated, this would be less frequently the case. Many physicians still also
end up working in, or managing, large private practices with complicated financial arrangements, but we know that proportionately fewer
physicians are going into private practice at present and that today's
generations of postresidency and fellowship doctors generally prefer to
be employed by large health systems. Finally, physicians clearly are potential targets for "get rich quick schemes," and some have a tendency
to make bad investment decisions.

The solution? Physicians need to be better financially educated than
they are at present, especially female physicians, and such education
should really be a lifelong activity, ideally starting prior to medical
school and continuing on past retirement. Financial competencies
should be integrated into the outcome competencies most medical
schools and residency programs now require. Better financially educated physicians are likely to be more productive and clinically successful during their careers. They will also be less personally stressed and
have fewer relationship problems in which, as Cathy and Brett described, finances are a massive stressor. A stronger financial setting and
plan also will allow physicians to make career choices that are not necessarily based on a short-term need to rapidly pay off debts, for instance. They would then be able to look beyond "lifestyle" specialties

that may not suit their passion and choose areas of medical expertise that really suit their personalities and long-term career preferences.

In conclusion, good financial knowledge and skills are an important component of the menu for any physician who wishes to avoid burnout and achieve professional and personal well-being. Just as education in personal relationships is key to the success of all physicians, so should financial knowledge and skills be part of every major physician education program.

References

American Medical Association Physician Communications Team: Why doctors marry doctors: exploring medical marriages. Resident and Student Health, January 3, 2019. Available at: https://www.ama-assn.org/residents-students/resident-student-health/why-doctors-marry-doctors-exploring-medical-marriages. Accessed May 25, 2019.

Arora H, Arora K: Six things we learned (and more) and dual-physician marriages. Physician Family, Winter 2018. Available at: https://bluetoad.com/publication/?i=469153andarticle_id=2986175andview=articleBrowser#{%22issue_id%22:469153,%22page%22:20}. Accessed May 25, 2019.

Association of American Medical Colleges: Debt, Costs and Loan Repayment Fact Card. Washington, DC, Association of American Medical Colleges, 2018. Available at: https://store.aamc.org/medical-student-education-debt-costs-and-loan-repayment-fact-card-2018-pdf.html. Accessed May 25, 2019.

Drummond D: The medical marriage: date night power tips and more. You Can Be a Happy MD (website), November 2014. Available at: https://www.thehappymd.com/blog/the-medical-marriage-date-night-secrets-and-more. Accessed May 25, 2019.

Gabbard GO, Menninger RW: Medical Marriages. Washington, DC, American Psychiatric Press, 1988

Hillin T: 13 simple tricks to a long and happy marriage. Huffington Post, October 6, 2014. Available at: https://www.huffpost.com/entry/happy-marriage-advice_n_5941372. Accessed May 26, 2019.

Kane L: Medscape Physician Wealth and Debt Report. Medscape (website), May 9, 2018. https://www.medscape.com/slideshow/2018-physician-wealth-debt-report-6009863. Accessed June 8, 2019.

Kane L: Medscape Public Health and Preventive Medicine Physician Lifestyle, Happiness and Burnout Report 2019. Medscape (website), February 20, 2019. Available at: https://www.medscape.com/slideshow/2019-lifestyle-public-health-6011057. Accessed May 25, 2019

Myers MF: Doctors' Marriages: A Look at the Problems and Their Solutions. Washington, DC, American Psychiatric Press, 1994

Sotile WM, Sotile MO: The Medical Marriage: Sustaining Healthy Relationships for Physicians and Their Families. Chicago, IL, American Medical Association, 2000

Chapter 10

THE JOY AND MEANING OF MEDICINE

Scenario

"It's amazing—I think I'm busier now that I'm retired than I was when I was working at the hospital. Look at all the preparation we've done for the Well-Being Advisory Board meeting next week! It all looks great. Thanks so much, Ellen."

Dr. Louise Newton smiled across the table in appreciation for all the hard work her colleague, Ellen Jackson, had completed. Louise looked around the well-furnished office. It was designed in a mixture of grays and blues, and the walls were adorned with matching steel-gray-framed pictures of several exotic tourist spots, including views of the Golden Gate and Brooklyn Bridges. Others showed various clinics and hospitals where members of the Hills Medical Society worked. A new, modern computer console sat atop a circular work desk in the center of the room that was surrounded by matching chairs.

Louise was looking forward to the meeting next week and thought all the preparations were in place. She stood up from her chair, took a deep breath, and stretched. A slim, conservatively dressed woman with short, sandy hair, today she wore a brown suit and matching silk scarf and her usual thin, gold-rimmed glasses. She looked the picture of fitness and health; acquaintances were often surprised to learn she was a retired pediatrician because she looked closer to 50 years old than to 60. She kept fit with regular hiking and played golf with a handicap of 15 that she knew she could improve if she could find time to play more than once per week. She could not see her handicap improving soon, however, because her life was so full with her volunteering and community activities. When she occasionally reflected on her professional life, she genuinely could not understand how she had had time to work as a full-time physician in the past. She knew she had made the right decision when she had finally retired from clinical work 3 years previously, after working part-time for a few years before.

Ellen Jackson, who had now been CEO[1] of the Society for nearly a decade, knew Louise well. She had worked with her on committees for years, but it was only during the past year, while Louise had been serving as president, that they had become friends. They had a mutual passion for working on behalf of the medical group that represented more than 6,000 physicians in the western region of the United States.

"I'm so pleased with the advisory group on physician well-being that we've put together and how enthusiastic everyone has been about this project," Ellen said. "I know that will be a longstanding legacy of yours, Louise. After all, you have driven this topic while you've been president, and you're such a great example of how physicians should look after themselves, their colleagues, and their community. I just wish you'd be more willing to tell your own story to inspire others."

Ellen knew she was taking a bit of a risk asking Louise again about this, because they had talked about it several times, and each time Louise had been adamant about preserving her privacy. However, she felt strongly that Louise was such a good example of resilience and overcoming adversity that her colleagues could learn so much from her.

"I know you want me to do that, and I know why. I really do want to help my colleagues as much as possible, and I've been thinking a lot about your request, Ellen. I wonder if it would be possible to talk about myself on a podcast, perhaps with a series of preplanned areas of discussion and the assurance that I can cut any sections I don't feel comfortable about? We didn't discuss that as an approach for telling my story, but I think a podcast might be okay with me if we do it carefully

---

[1]CEO=chief executive officer.

and find a sensitive interviewer. I was impressed by the example podcast you played for me last week; it was like hearing a friend's life story in my living room."

Louise looked at Ellen, who smiled back. Ellen was pleased by her friend's gradual change of mind, but she was not at all surprised. Ellen had a comprehensive program on well-being planned for the Society and knew that Louise was the right person to be the medical leader and example for other physicians. She thought about the first time she had sat down with Louise to discuss her idea for a physician well-being program that would be available to—and, she hoped, would involve—most of the physicians in her region, whether they belonged to the Society or not. She knew, as did almost all of the regional physicians, about Louise's tragic background. Louise's husband, who had been a prominent obstetrician, and both of her teenage daughters had been killed by a methamphetamine-intoxicated hit-and-run driver 15 years previously. Louise had been badly injured but had recovered from her crushed pelvis and broken legs, although her psychological injuries were much more severe. Ellen knew Louise still had regular nightmares and continued to see a local psychiatrist who specialized in treating physicians and who, Ellen had discovered, was helping a surprising number of the medical society members. She had recruited him for her advisory board early on.

Ellen pushed her thick, blonde hair back, using her glasses as a headband. She decided it was time to relax. Ellen took pride in looking her best and keeping fit. At 5'8" tall, she was able to stand out well in her new pink linen blouse, classic navy suit, and 3-inch heels. Her simple gold wedding band was a reminder of her long, successful marriage that was perfect in all respects except for the lack of children, something she always shrugged off in polite conversation. She turned to Louise.

"Well, I have to say I'm pleased by your change of mind, Louise. I should probably show you the draft agenda for next week's meeting. I want to go over it with you." Smiling, she passed Louise the sheet of paper. "There, look at item one. The creation of more regular podcasts featuring members discussing their own view of well-being in medicine. I've been hoping for a while that you would be the interviewer for the first few, but now I'm wondering if you would be prepared to be the first person interviewed. Is that a possibility?"

"How do you do it, Ellen? I think you've had all this planned. I can't believe how good you are at getting people to do what you want!" Louise exclaimed, not sure whether to be flattered or embarrassed. She certainly wasn't angry, although she could see how effectively Ellen had manipulated her to get what she wanted. "I knew I should never have become friends with you. You know me too well, I suspect, and knew that I'd eventually agree to do what you wanted. Oh well, you win."

Ellen laughed. "Okay, so maybe I outmaneuvered you, but I also know that you will only allow yourself to be manipulated if you want to be. Anyway, let's face it: Even if you tell only half of your story, I think you will help a great number of your colleagues." She slowed down her talk and looked seriously at Louise. "I know you won't want to talk about the crash and losing Bruce and the girls. I'm not suggesting that. What I do think would be helpful is discussing your whole approach to practicing medicine—your outside activities, especially volunteering, and your concept of giving, and how all that ultimately led to your retirement from clinical practice. I leave it to you to decide how much you want to share about your background. To me, your approach to your life is what will help our local physicians. After all, you're a classic Baby Boomer, just like a third of our members, and you've shown others the way to transition out of practice. You wouldn't believe how many are having difficulty doing that and come to us for advice. They want to know about so many issues—taking up new interests, financial management, finding colleagues with interests in common whom they can get to know, working part-time, or volunteering. They need help making their lives feel more interesting and meaningful."

Louise nodded. "I know physicians need to learn about retiring and how to transition out of clinical practice, but I didn't realize you thought I had done this so well. Thank you for that; I really appreciate what you said. What is it that you think I can teach others? I'm always so afraid that if I speak publicly about anything personal that I will be expected to talk about the crash, and I prefer not to do that. I've spent enough time working through it in private, and those memories and feelings I prefer to keep to myself."

"I know that only too well, Louise," Ellen answered empathetically. "Let's just have you talk about the past 10 years of your life. Do you know what struck me first about you when we started to get to know each other a few years ago?"

"No. That I was single? That I was looking to do things with the Society? That everyone used to look at me sympathetically but never said anything about my losses? Embarrassed and not sure how to speak to me?"

"Maybe a bit of all of those. You're right. It never ceases to amaze me how difficult many doctors find it to be open with you. How they sometimes, even now, treat you with kid gloves because they all know what you've been through. It surprises me that as doctors they don't have the communication skills with a colleague to show empathy but at the same time to be respectful of your privacy. I think that's one of the things you can teach them, if you want, although it's not what I'd planned: how to approach a colleague in distress respectfully and tactfully."

"I think not," Louise replied. "I also think I should keep away from substances and driving, which is just as much a problem for some doctors, especially with alcohol, as it is for the general population. I'm still too angry about that and wouldn't trust myself on that topic. So what do you think I've done well, Ellen? And please do tell me what it was you noticed about me early on. We seem to have gotten off that track."

"It was your approach to giving and volunteering, how you were so genuine and active about it and seemed to really enjoy the work. I remember you telling me that you'd discovered you looked forward to the 2 half-days of volunteering you were doing at the time more than you enjoyed your clinical practice, but you never told me why that was. Can you remember your first volunteer jobs? I think one was at the women's shelter and one was at the local primary school. Is that correct?"

Louise smiled; those were happy memories. "Yes, you're right. Those were my first two volunteer roles. You know, I did both of them for several years, and I still go back to the school to do some basic biology seminars with the sixth graders before they leave for middle school."

"What did you do there? Why did you enjoy it so much?"

"Well, not surprisingly, the roles were very different, but they both involved direct contact with children, so I thought I could use my pediatric skills but not have the administrative restrictions of medical practice. At the shelter, I was referred a lot of children. Many of them had been through awful traumas, some not unlike my own, really. What I liked was being able to spend lots of time with them without being limited by a schedule. I've always liked talking to children. I learned a lot about play therapy from one of the social workers there. It was fascinating watching the children paint, draw, and play while they talked about their worries, their fun, their families, and their fears. I'd never really taken the time to do that with children before; I'd always left it to the social workers and child psychiatrists. I suddenly found a whole new area of work that I loved, and I think I actually did help quite a few of the children. I especially liked the younger ones, below the age of 6, because they were so open about everything. Some of them asked a lot about me too, and I gradually found I could tell them about some of my losses, which in retrospect was helpful. Once I even ended up painting pictures of my own children in response to the inquisition of a particularly sweet 5-year-old whose older siblings had been murdered. I thought of trying to retrain and take a fellowship in child psychiatry, but it hit me that one of the main reasons I really enjoyed this work was because I was less restricted by professional boundaries. I loved being able to just spend time with the children. It was freeing for me and made me think about the way I was practicing clinically. The answer seemed to be to change my clinical practice style rather than try to get a new qualification, so that's what I did."

"How fascinating. What did that involve?" said Ellen.

"Well, it made me turn my practice into one where I could give more time when a patient required it. I completely changed my business model and got away from the restrictions and stress of billing codes. I was a bit ahead of my time, but I developed a pediatric concierge practice. I wasn't so worried about the financial side because Bruce had been well insured, but it worked out well; I told all of my patients' families that I would be charging a monthly retainer for my services and joined up with an adult concierge practice so that we could help cover each other. I ended up being able to see my patients as much as was necessary and found my work so much more satisfying. I was in control of my practice and no longer involved with the insurance companies. I loved it, and so did my patients. My concierge practice allowed me take on a reasonable panel size, and I could decide who needed 10 versus 45 minutes. Most pediatric appointments don't require 30-plus minutes, but when that was needed, I could manage it. The parents and the kids liked it, and so did I. I never had problems getting referrals, and the practice was the best of all worlds for me and the families I worked with. I was less stressed and was enjoying medicine and my life in general."

"Well done! But what about the school volunteering? It seems that you've continued that all these years," said Ellen.

"That's true, but now I teach a 10-week course once per year on human anatomy and physiology, really preparing the sixth graders for what they will start learning about puberty and their bodies in middle school. In the past, I'd worked mainly with children in the first and second grades, helping in the classroom, not really trying to use my medical skills. I wasn't there as a physician. Yet I really wasn't completely divorced from it, especially with the children who had ADHD[2] or autism who often had behavioral problems. I was really a teacher's aide one afternoon per week for several years, and I specialized in teaching them art. I studied up and became an art docent for 5- and 6-year-olds. It was fascinating for me. I was given a large container of prints each week to share

---

[2]ADHD = attention-deficit/hyperactivity disorder.

with the children, and they became so engaged! They liked being shown famous paintings and being encouraged to tell everyone, including me, what they thought about the art in front of them. Then we would bring out the art supplies, and I would encourage them to draw or paint as they wished—no rules. I enjoyed seeing how they expressed themselves in art class and watching them develop over the course of a year.

"I learned a lot about art, and art history, and I used to love hearing how the children interpreted famous paintings. You should've seen their fascination with Mona Lisa's eyes and how they seemed to move and follow people around. They made up the most fantastic explanatory stories for this. One creative boy suggested she might have been a zombie on *The Walking Dead*. What an influence TV has!"

"But you've been going there for more than 12 years by now, I suspect. How did your role change?" said Ellen.

"It's sad to say, but ultimately it changed because of the school's funding situation and their need for a biology teacher. I was available and free, and the principal approached me to take up part of this role. So about 3 years ago I changed from art docent to biology teacher. I enjoy what I do, but it's a bit more formal, and I'm not sure I'll continue for too long. I feel I had a better relationship with the children when I could communicate with them through the paint box."

"Tell me what you've been doing since you gave up your clinical practice. How was it, making that change?"

"Giving up my practice was the big decision. I had been working 3–4 days per week for a number of years and doing the volunteering and playing some golf the rest of the time. Remember, I was still recovering from losing Bruce and the girls, so I didn't want lots of extra pressure, and I was suddenly a single woman at a time when I'd been expecting a meaningful retirement with my family. I think at one level I was still overwhelmed with my losses, or at least that's what my psychiatrist thought. I was clinging to my clinical practice to provide some structure in my life, as though it were a life raft. For me, the problem was letting go of that life raft and the security of clinical practice. I think that's what a lot of physicians find after practicing for 30 years or more. It can be pretty scary to suddenly stop. What do you do instead? I was lucky because I was financially secure and had a good financial advisor, so I didn't need to worry about that."

Ellen nodded. "It's amazing how many physicians are bad money managers and don't plan ahead for their retirement. For intelligent people, it's really very odd. Perhaps they're just used to assuming that if they continue to work hard everything will work out okay. What I see at the Society is that every time we put on a financial planning seminar we're inundated, and not only with the young doctors. A surprising number of your more mature colleagues attend."

"You're right. That's something I will always be grateful to Bruce for. He was very organized, and he left me financially secure after he died." Louise suddenly looked away from Ellen, feeling emotional and distressed. "I don't know why that suddenly hit me, but I guess this grief process just goes on a long time. I'm sorry if I'm embarrassing you."

"Don't worry. It's good to see you show some emotion sometimes, Louise. You are one of those women whom everyone finds rather intimidating because of your amazing capacity to overcome difficulties and to show resilience in the face of whatever life throws at you. I know you're good at acting positively even when you're feeling down," Ellen replied sympathetically.

Louise wiped her eyes with a tissue and gathered herself. "Where was I? The decision to retire, that's right. Well, I had three main reasons. First and most importantly, I thought that after 34 years as a pediatrician, I had done my bit. My passion for my children and their families was less than it used to be, and I deserved a break. I started looking around for other things to do and was enjoying my volunteering more than working as a physician, where much of the work, even in a concierge practice, was pretty simple. Second, Bruce and I had always talked about retiring at around 60 years old so we could travel and work on our 'bucket list,' and when I discovered that the average physician worked until they were 68 years old, I knew that wasn't for me and that I would finish earlier. I wanted to see if I could enjoy myself again after losing my family. It really hit me when I realized that I would never be a grandmother because both of my daughters had died—that my losses and grief would continue, even vicariously, going forward. I knew that Bruce would have wanted me to give myself some time." Louise paused and looked out the window, deep in thought. She was remembering Bruce, the love of her life, and still missed him deeply.

"What was the third reason? It sounds like you already had two strong motives," Ellen said, trying to bring her friend out of her reverie.

"I did, but the tipping point came one day when I was here for a committee meeting. I don't think I've ever told you this. Do you remember Abbie Parsons, that sweet, young internal medicine physician who was quite an active member here for several years?"

"Yes, I do; she was very friendly but quiet. She moved away from here about 3 years ago, I think. I was always surprised at her move because she seemed so keen to get to know everyone. I had coffee with her several times right at this table."

"Well, she had another side, and she confided in me about it one day. She told me she had severe bipolar disorder and a tendency to self-medicate when she was sick. She apparently had almost lost her license on several occasions when she was manic. Fortunately, she had enough insight not to practice when she was unwell, but the medical board still became involved after a hospital reported her for stealing tranquilizers, and they were reviewing her fitness to practice. At her request I tried to help her and keep her practicing, but she decided it was all too difficult, and when she became depressed about 3 years ago, rather than fight the medical board, she just gave in and voluntarily gave up her medical license. She resisted treatment and always refused to go to a physician health program. It was awful, because she used me as her main shoulder to cry on. Her husband was hopeless; he was a nice guy but had no insight. A building contractor, he was quite successful and was supportive of her when she was first ill, but he just didn't understand the professional requirements needed to continue practicing. He eventually left her, taking their two young children with him when she was hospitalized on one occasion. In the end, she literally took flight. She left the area and returned to the East Coast to live with her parents. They had always been her main support when she was younger, and she reverted to them in this crisis. I kept in touch for a while, but for the past year she hasn't been taking my calls or responding to my e-mails, so I really don't know what's happening with her. I hope she isn't in big trouble. It always used to worry me that she might attempt suicide, but I haven't heard anything, and I think her parents would contact me if something like that happened."

"I'm so sorry. I had no idea. That's tragic. It must've been kept very quiet, because I heard nothing about all this," said Ellen.

"I guess that's because, as you know, there's this 'cone of silence' about impaired doctors," said Louise. "Anyway Abbie had a big impact on me and made me think that I could really do something worthwhile with my medical knowledge and experience that was not centered on pediatrics. So that was my tipping point, the reason I finally decided to retire. I wanted to contribute to the health of my colleagues, and that's why I've become so much more involved in the Society and in trying to get our 'Joy and Meaning in Medicine' program going. For me, this is a new passion, and something I can do on a volunteer basis, that is even more meaningful than my previous clinical career. So Abbie was good for me; she made my decision to retire much easier. She gave me a reason to look at alternative useful ways to enjoy myself and to do good, which is so much more rewarding than I could ever have expected."

"How fascinating!" Ellen smiled broadly at Louise. "See, I told you that you would be great on our podcast. Wait 'til our members hear how you got interested in physician well-being and how rewarding it is."

"Okay, okay, I give in! I'll coordinate a time to record it with your assistant—as long as I'm primarily able to promote the 'Joy and Meaning in Medicine' program. And of course I won't mention any specifics that would identify Abbie."

One month later, Louise recorded her interview for the podcast.

"Let me tell you what we have planned for the program that we're calling 'Joy and Meaning in Medicine,'" said Louise. She smiled at her interviewer, a family medicine physician who was becoming somewhat of a local celebrity through his own social media involvement promoting the importance of preventive medicine. "We have several components, all of which overlap, and that we hope will reduce the amount of burnout and distress common in many physicians."

"This sounds really important, Dr. Newton. Like many physicians, I suffered burnout in a past job, but now, having changed my work to focus much more on prevention and a community approach to medicine, I believe I have left that behind. Am I an example of the sort of doctors you are trying to help?" Dr. Anthony Read moved his face to the side of his condenser microphone to catch Louise's eye fully, making it clear that he was serious about his personal question.

"You know, Dr. Read, I had no idea you'd experienced burnout, but given that the problem is so common, it's not surprising. So yes, you *are* an example of a colleague we'd like to assist and involve. I'd like to pick up your comments about a community approach to medicine, because that's exactly what we're planning for this program. As you know, most burnout is caused by organizational and systemic stress. It's not usually the fault of physicians, who are mostly very resilient people. Recent research shows that medical students, at entry to medical school, are actually more resilient than nonmedical postgrads, but 10 years later are twice as burned out as their professional nonmedical equivalents in the population. So we're taking a series of approaches aimed at changing the organization and culture of the local medical system as well as putting in place programs to help doctors rediscover their resilience skills."

"That sounds great. Before we get on to why you became involved in setting up this program, perhaps you could summarize what it involves? I really like the emphasis on changing the culture of medicine. I know I've secretly always felt a bit ashamed that became burned out. It sounds like one of the first approaches might be education for all of us about not blaming ourselves, about not blaming the doctor. Is that the case?"

"You know, it certainly is," responded Louise. "I'm pleased to hear you say that. Setting up this program has really made me think about our lives as physicians. I imagine you're similar to me. I remember how, when I started medical school, I felt like I was on top of the world and could conquer any problem. I went to medical school to spend time with patients, to cure them, certainly not to spend several hours each day filling in forms and sitting at a computer. I was positive, resilient, and used to working hard and playing hard. I thought every problem, no matter how difficult, could be solved if I just put my mind to it."

"That's right. I can well remember the thrill of starting medical school. I had the most enthusiastic classmates. Is that something you're hoping to recapture with this program?"

"Most certainly. That's why we've called it 'Joy and Meaning in Medicine,' because we know that's how physicians start their careers, and I personally believe that it's possible to recapture that essence. But we need to work at it, because so many forces in health care fight against us. For example, I have never met a doctor who said he or she went to medical school to be able to spend massive amounts of time documenting notes in the EMR![3]"

"Well, that is certainly true," said a thoughtful Dr. Read. "Let's get back to what you are doing, though?"

"Well, we have activities both for individuals and for groups of physicians. One example is our series of evening seminars and socials that starts shortly. It will include everything from painting, writing, and food and wine appreciation to financial management, volunteering, public speaking, and leadership skills. These will not be your typical lecture-style evenings; for instance, we're combining public speaking and wine appreciation by inviting a speaker from Toastmasters to co-present with a sommelier from one of our best restaurants. We intend these evenings to be very interactive and hope that they will engage our members in a positive way so that they not only learn things of use and interest to them but also, just as importantly, network and get to know their colleagues. We're going to hold these evenings at all sorts of different places—restaurants, art galleries, wineries—almost anywhere that is *not* medical. In fact, that networking issue is something we think is super important, especially for those doctors who work for different health systems and would not normally get to know each other. So we're also setting up some monthly 'at home' events for physicians who live in differing geograph-

---

[3]EMR=electronic medical record.

ical areas where they can get to know each other better and gain more in-dividual support. We're even paying for psychologists to go to each of these meetings to facilitate the groups as they get going."

"That sounds excellent—networking *and* fun. I like the sound of the painting and writing evenings and will check them out. But what else do you have?"

"Naturally, we've set up a website where everything is listed, and that has a well-being blog and provides access to what I hope will be-come a regular series of podcasts, just like this one we're doing now. We're fortunate that so many of our physicians have such interesting backgrounds. It isn't really hard to find people to interview who have fascinating stories. You'd be surprised by how many doctors like the idea of doing exactly what you're doing now, being guest podcast interview-ers. Our next podcast features Dr. Nigel Hawley, who, before he went to medical school and trained as a cardiac surgeon, was not only in the Ma-rines as a special services soldier but also completed a master's degree in philosophy. Now, in the latter stages of his career, as he starts to wind down his operating room time, he has become the chief wellness officer for his health system. So we'll have lots to discuss with him. Setting up these podcasts has been a great exercise in finding out just how diverse are the interests and backgrounds of many of our local physicians."

Louise stopped for a moment. She was keen to pause and change di-rection. She looked across the interview table above the bulbous micro-phones toward Dr. Read, who, like her, was wearing large high-fidelity earphones. "Of course, we're doing a lot more than just education and networking. We're also offering serious services for those physicians who want to take them up, including an anonymous self-assessment survey on our website that allows individuals to self-stratify themselves on the basis of their degrees of risk of depression, substance use disor-der, and suicidality. We employ a psychologist to review all the results, and she engages with the respondents whose survey results show them at high risk to offer help if they are prepared to break their anonymity, either seeing them herself or arranging for their referral to other mental health professionals. We're finding this to be a great way of getting over our doctors' traditional reticence to engage in care themselves."

"That's fascinating. I've heard of such self-assessment tools being used in other health systems occasionally as a way of engaging high-risk physicians in care," said Dr. Read. "What else have you been doing?"

"Well, we've been following up on a regional burnout survey that we undertook a few months ago that showed that up to 40% of our phy-sicians had some symptoms of burnout. I'm proud to say that we've managed to get grant funding for up to six coaching sessions each for a large number of our members who are interested. We have several accredited life coaches working for us, all of whom are expert in burnout and similar stresses, and we already have more than 20 physicians signed up for the sessions via our website. Of course, if they want more than six sessions, they can arrange that themselves, in which case they pay for the extra sessions. We hope that this coaching will be sufficient for most of our members, but we know that some have more significant problems such as depression and substance abuse. Of course, we also know physicians have an increased risk of suicide, so what we have done for those doctors is arrange a process whereby they can be referred urgently to psychiatrists in our community who have volunteered to see colleagues and to fast track any referrals from our program."

Dr. Read, who'd been listening intently throughout and letting his excellent interviewee have her head, decided it was time to intervene and present some ideas of his own. He thought the conversation was important and had just come to the conclusion that he felt safe enough to reveal some of his more deeply hidden secrets.

"Dr. Newton, all that you're doing is so important. It seems to me that you've set up a substantial range of coaching and counseling services that are specifically designed for physicians. And that's on top of all the education and networking opportunities you're offering your members! I wish all this had been available 20 years ago when I first came here. I've never spoken about this in public before, but I am one of the people who could have really benefited from this program. I seriously contemplated suicide after my first marriage broke up and my now ex-wife took my children away. I was lucky and had some very supportive friends who made sure I was well looked after and treated, so I did fine in the end, but this program is such a great way to reduce the stigma of psychiatric disorders. That shame and stigma kept me from initially getting help, and since then I can think of at least two colleagues whom I believe died from suicide, although one died in a single-vehicle accident and the coroner did not determine it to be intentional. It's great that these sorts of services are being made available. I just hope they get used. Congratulations on setting up this program. What a great role for a regional medical society to play."

Commentary

Two major themes of importance are discussed in this scenario. The first is retirement and how physicians can transition into this role in a way that not only allows them to contribute meaningfully to society, if they so choose, but also to take up the role as a respected elder within the medical and broader community. One approach to retirement involves volunteering and taking alternative roles that enable physicians to use their skills and experience to benefit their communities, just as Louise did. The second theme is the need for comprehensive programs that encourage the continued well-being and health of communities of physicians, like the one Ellen and Louise were developing in the regional medical society. The programs described in this scenario are based on those developed and run by the Sierra Sacramento Valley Medical Society (SSVMS; www.ssvms.org), which is a national leader in this field. The SSVMS has developed a truly innovative role and set of programs for its physician community and their families that could be copied and continuously enhanced by other medical societies nationally.

So what do we know about physicians and retirement? Overall, surprisingly little has been written on this topic, and almost no formal studies exist, so the first conclusion has to be that this is yet another area for physician well-being that merits considerable research. It is actually quite difficult to determine the precise age of retirement of many physicians. Is it retirement from full-time practice? From part-time practice? From paid or unpaid practice? From teaching and research, as opposed to clinical work? However, quite a lot of interesting information, usually anecdotal, has been written in blogs and presented in podcasts that provides valuable insights.

What we do know is that the median age of retirement from clinical activities by primary care physicians is 65 years (Petterson et al. 2016). The retirement age from clinical activities varies by specialty, and several studies have shown variations ranging from about 64.5 years for obstetrician-gynecologists up to 66.5 years for cardiologists. Women tend to retire 1 year earlier than men, but many physicians continue to be active in other professional, nonclinical activities after retirement, and the median age of retirement from all professional activities is typically about 1 year later, at 66 years, although this is likely younger than in the past, as the American Academy of Family Physicians has reported that the average age of physician retirement was 70 in 1980 (The Physicians Foundation 2016). This is in comparison with the average age of retirement of the non-physician workforce of 63 years. Data are lacking as to how many physicians work part-time prior to retirement.

But why do physicians eventually decide to retire, and why later than other professionals? An interesting blog by *Wall Street Physician* (2018) examined this and described a series of financially oriented reasons, which I have adapted as follows:

1. *Age.* Many individuals simply pick a preferred age and retire at that time, even if they have not reached their financial goals. They decide to have a less stressful lifestyle on the basis that time is a nonrenewable resource.
2. *Net worth.* Many physicians have a target financial retirement number in mind and retire when they have reached it.
3. *Ability/Health.* Medicine is a difficult profession and is constantly changing, as described throughout this book. It is hard to keep up with the latest literature and new drugs, treatments, and technologies. This leads many physicians to retire before they lose their abilities or the capacity to keep current. The EMR is one reason that substantial numbers of physicians have retired over the past decade. Other physicians retire because of impaired health, and it is fairly uncommon, for instance, to find surgeons operating full time beyond the age of 63.

Wall Street Physician gives the following advice: "Don't be like the professional athlete when it comes to retirement….The goal is to do it on your own terms. Athletes are notorious for staying in the game for too long…even though their skills have noticeably declined." The author concluded that financial independence gives physicians the option to retire on their own terms, so one message for all physicians is to ensure they obtain good financial advice from experts as early in their career as possible, ideally starting in medical school, so that they can control their own retirement decisions, just as Louise did in the scenario (Wall Street Physician 2018). Many physicians find it genuinely hard to retire simply because medicine is such a meaningful, all-enveloping occupation that they do not wish to give up the role. This has been well described by Mokotoff (2018), who, in an insightful blog titled "Why Doctors Don't Like to Retire," wrote the following:

> I believe there are multiple reasons. For many physicians, medicine is the only employment they have had in their adult life. Despite drops in salaries and autonomy, they still enjoy above-average wealth and income and may fear loss of this post-retirement…. Some have few hobbies and fear boredom. That is a reasonable concern. Most of us are used to being respected by the public and inwardly fear that loss as well…. [T]he act of retirement brings into hard focus that this is indeed the "last stage" of one's life. Although we deal with the death and dying of our patients daily, when it is "our" death and dying, well, that is a different matter. The hassles of corporate and industrialized medicine will continue to affect physician retirement rates. However, for many of those in the profession, the idea of life without medicine is just too scary to contemplate.

When physicians finally do retire, either completely or partially, most live a rewarding and interesting life, just as Louise did in the scenario. Fawcett (2018) recently described some discoveries he made during his first year of retirement:

- I don't miss medicine…. I think tapering off my practice, while I started a new writing, speaking, blogging, consulting business, played a big part in allowing me to let go of this major part of my life….
- Vacationing feels different now. When I was working as a surgeon, I needed vacation time to get away and unwind. Now I live a much more relaxed life, and I don't need to get away to unwind. Now when I travel, it is for a different purpose, to explore the world. I changed my perspective from unwinding to exploring, and that is a whole different feeling. I also write while on vacation…. It is almost like a reversal now. When I'm home, I'm on vacation, and then I go away on vacation to get some work done….
- I'm never going to catch up. I did have some big hopes for catching up on a lot of things that were getting put off. The state of caught up doesn't exist….
- My life is very good now and much more relaxed. I'm glad I pulled the trigger on repurposing, as I feel I have a new mission in life and am enjoying its pursuit. Letting go of the old life was easier than I thought.

In retirement, many physicians "give back" to their communities by volunteering or using their skills for the benefit of everyone, as Louise was doing. The Medical Board of California, for instance, maintains a Volunteer Physician Registry (www.mbc.ca.gov/VPR). The Board allows retired physicians to retain their medical licenses at no cost if they are doing volunteer or *pro bono* work only and encourages all physicians via the registry to give back to their communities. Physicians can sign up and indicate the type of volunteer work they are interested in doing as well as detail other important facts, such as their specialty skills and language capacities. The registry also allows groups such as clinics for the underserved, schools, shelters, and charities to search for volunteer physicians, performing an important matching role.

Numerous other volunteer positions are available for physicians, whether retired or not, especially working for medical societies and professional organizations nationally and internationally. Many of these organizations would be unable to fulfill their goals if physician volunteers were not available to take up workforce, committee, and board positions. Putting the search term "volunteer physician" into

Google returns innumerable opportunities, including several groups whose primary purpose is to place volunteer health providers from many disciplines into positions around the world, as well as throughout the United States. Meszaros (2018) reviewed the benefits of medical volunteering and concluded that helping others is good for the human soul and can help reignite one's passion for medical practice. Among the many benefits of volunteerism for both mind and body Meszaros described were counteracting the effects of stress, anger, anxiety, burnout, and depression; increasing self-confidence; providing a sense of purpose; protecting against cognitive and physical decline; connecting with others; advancing a career; and bringing fun and fulfillment.

Of course, not all doctors wish to take up volunteer positions, preferring a change of career using their medical degree as a core requirement of their new paid position. Although I have highlighted several such opportunities in these chapters, often involving telemedicine technologies and working from home for clinical or consulting work, many other careers are available for those physicians who do not wish to continue with clinical work for whatever reason. The extent of these options is beyond the scope of this book, but they tend to include positions involving writing or data analysis on health topics in the fields of media, insurance, finance, and technology. When taken up in retirement, as in this scenario, this work tends to have the added bonus of improving our "healthspan" rather than our "lifespan" by maintaining our resilience through engagement with life and maintaining our cognitive and physical function, both of which are essential for successful aging.

The final theme concerns the innovative solutions that regional medical societies, associations, or groups can implement across their often geographically diverse communities. Visit the SSVMS website (www.ssvms.org) and explore the "Joy of Medicine" program on which much of this scenario is based (www.joyofmedicine.org). Since 1860, the SSVMS has brought together physicians to promote the health and well-being of physicians and the patients they serve. With more than 5,500 physician members in the Sacramento region, SSVMS provides advocacy, programs, and services to promote access to quality medical care and to help physicians reclaim the joy of practicing medicine. The leadership of SSVMS, a not-for-profit professional organization, understands the struggles physicians face on a daily basis. "SSVMS is passionate about helping physicians find joy and fulfillment in the profession of medicine," says SSVMS CEO Aileen Wetzel. "Our goal is to engage physicians, medical groups and health system leaders in a long-term conversation that will help physicians recognize the signs of burnout, build meaningful resilience, and promote systemic improvements that help physicians thrive" (personal communication, May 20, 2019).

The Joy of Medicine program describes its vision thus: "The Joy of Medicine will relieve physician pain and help to reclaim the joy of practicing medicine through education, advocacy and program services designed to nurture individual well-being and collegiality and to promote systems-wide changes."

SSVMS' Joy of Medicine Advisory Committee includes medical group leaders and physician wellness champions from all local medical groups as well as physicians in private practice and medical students from two local schools. The committee meets every other month, sharing best practices and advising SSVMS on the creation and sustainability of the various components of the program. The program itself, funded in part by external collaborators as detailed on its website, consists of nine specific services, several of which are also described in the scenario. These services are described in the following list and are adapted from the Joy of Medicine website (www.joyofmedicine.org):

1. Access to up to six sponsored "resiliency consultations" through self-referral with a vetted licensed psychologist or life coach that focus on assisting physicians with burnout and practice or personal problems
2. Physician peer-groups that meet monthly in physicians' homes to provide communal support and to enable physicians who live in the same geographical area to discuss the challenges and successes of being a physician
3. Psychiatric consultation, with rapid urgent assessments from psychiatrists experienced in treating physicians as patients, for any physician who self-refers through the program
4. Biannual physician surveys on needs, stressors, burnout, and possible solutions, with results fed back to all local health systems and published in white papers
5. Monthly Joy of Medicine "on-call" podcasts, available through iTunes, that focus on the lives of local physicians and how they maintain their own well-being
6. Gratitude popups where staff from SSVMS attend meetings and lectures at local hospitals to personally thank physicians for what they do, as well as to give them small wellness-focused handouts, gifts, and raffle tickets
7. Online wellness library for physicians and medical students

8. Annual summit conference that typically attracts up to 200 physicians for about 4 hours of interactive talks and fast-paced "lightning rounds" of short topical presentations
9. Physician socials and seminars on a wide range of topics for individuals and families, ranging from movie nights for the family to financial wellness seminars

Between them, this slate of offerings helps educate students and physicians on relevant topics, many of which are described in this book. It also provides networking and a social medical community for physicians and their families, seeks and implements specific solutions for burnout and stress, and offers nonstigmatizing ways for physicians to obtain individual and group counseling and support as well as formal psychiatric treatment if required. The SSVMS offers these services to all physicians in the region and breaks down the silos of individual health systems by crossing and involving all of them in a noncompetitive manner. Not surprisingly, many physicians have commented that it is both interesting and less threatening to discuss their work situations with physicians who primarily work in other health systems or environments and that they feel safer and less stigmatized in this style of setting. A large number of local physicians, initially taken aback at being thanked for their work at the "popups," have also learned the importance of gratitude and its positive impact on those receiving the thanks.

Other medical societies are considering setting up a similar range of services to SSVMS. I hope that they do so, because many of the group and individual services provided in this way are clearly less stigmatizing and less threatening to physicians than if they were provided by the physicians' own systems. The development of programs like the Joy of Medicine is an innovative solution to the stigma of burnout and distress felt by physicians.

References

Fawcett C: 6 things this physician learned after retiring. KevinMD.com, April 20, 2018. Available at: https://www.kevinmd.com/blog/2018/04/6-things-this-physician-learned-after-retiring.html. Accessed June 15, 2019.

Meszaros L: Physician volunteerism: The surprising benefits for doctors who do it. MDLinx, October 18, 2018. Available at: https://www.mdlinx.com/internal-medicine/article/2841 Accessed June 15, 2019.

Mokotoff D: Why physicians don't like to retire. KevinMD.com, August 19, 2018. Available at: https://www.kevinmd.com/blog/2018/08/why-doctors-dont-like-to-retire.html. Accessed June 15, 2019.

Petterson SM, Rayburn WF, Liaw WR: When Do Primary Care Physicians Retire? Implications for Workforce Projections. Ann Fam Med 14(4):344–349, 2016 27401422

The Physicians Foundation: 2016 Survey of America's Physicians: Practice Patterns and Perspectives. Columbia, SC, The Physicians Foundation, 2016. Available at: https://physiciansfoundation.org/wp-content/uploads/2018/01/Biennial_Physician_Survey_2016.pdf. Accessed June 15, 2019.

Wall Street Physician: Physician retirement age: when is the right time to retire? Wall Street Physician, January 10, 2018. Available at: http://www.wallstreetphysician.com/physician-retirement-age. Accessed June 15, 2019.

INDEX

Page numbers printed in **boldface** type refer to tables and figures.

AAMC. *See* Association of American Medical Colleges
ACA. *See* Affordable Care Act
ACEs. *See* Adverse childhood experiences
ACE Scale, 114, 120–121
  summary of, 121–122
Addiction
  in residents, 149–168
  treatment for, 160–162, 164–165
Adverse childhood experiences (ACEs), 114
Affordable Care Act (ACA), xvi
Alcohol abuse disorder, 203
  in physicians, xii
Allegheny College, 116
Alpha Omega Alpha Honor Medical Society, 20, 21–22
AMCAS. *See* American Medical College Admission Service
American College of Endocrinology, 83
American College of Physicians, 21
American Medical College Admission Service (AMCAS), 107
American Medical Students Association, 141

American Medical Women's Association, 92
Americans with Disabilities Act, 48–49
American Telemedicine Association, 87, 88
Anzia, Joan, 15–18
Arora, Dr., 99
Arora, Hans, 209–211
Arora, Kavita, 209–211
Association of American Medical Colleges (AAMC), 130
  perspective on clinician well-being, 145
  review of social media and application to medical school, 119–120

Baby Boomers, xvii, 24
Balint, Michael, 190
Beneficence, 17
Blogs
  on decision to retire, 228–230
  on health care about UCH, 28, 41–42
Brucer, Dr., 150
Burnout
  behavioral components of, 174–175
  detection of early signs of, 165
  of physicians, xv, 42

Burnout *(continued)*
  reduction of, xvii
  stigma attached to symptoms of,
    173–174
  symptoms of, 43, 88–89, 156
  technology for prevention of, 86
Burtone, Dr., 40
"Busy work." *See also* Electronic
  medical record (EMR)
  of physicians, xiv
  reduction of, xiv–xv

Canter, Marty, 193–214
Carbon dioxide emissions
  changes in, 186–188
Carbon Neutrality Initiative, 187
Careers
  alternative, in medicine, 185–186
  defining meaning in, 169–190
  medical marriages, 193–214
  medical specialty decisions, 213
  physician fulfillment and, 188–189
Carney, Mr., 29–30
Carnicle, Jocelyn, 118
Case vignettes
  of addiction in residents
    commentary, 162–167
    scenario, 149–162
  on biases and a well-being curric-
    ulum in medical school
    commentary, 140–146
    scenario, 125–139
  on cognitive dissonance and de-
    fining meaning in medicine
    commentary, 184–190
    scenario, 169–184
  on the culture of medicine,
    xviii–xix
    commentary, 15–25
    scenario, 1–15
  on health care
    blogs, 28, 41–42
    commentary, 42–50
    scenario, 27–42

    University City Health and,
      27–52
  of joy and meaning in medicine
    commentary, 227–233
    scenario, 215–227
  of medical marriages
    commentary, 207–214
    scenario, 193–206
  on morale in a clinical setting
    commentary, 69–76
    scenario, 53–69
  of pre-med vulnerability and
    trauma, 101–124
    commentary, 114–123
    scenario, 101–113
  on resilience
    commentary, 69–76
    scenario, 53–69
  on trust, mentoring, and
    innovation
    commentary, 91–99
    scenario, 77–91
Chief Wellness Officer (CWO)
  appointment of, 42
  description of, 46
  responsibilities of, 46–47
Childcare, 208–209
Chofan, Asim, 149–167
Cleveland Clinic, xv
Clinical services, 187
Cognitive dissonance, defining meaning in medicine and, 169–190
Collaboration, 97
Commitment, as attribute for successful entry into medical
  school, 118–119
Communication. *See also* Case
  vignettes
  as attribute for successful entry
    into medical school, 115
  in the health care industry, 33
  "phone tag," **97**
  with physicians, 70
  skills for, 219
  via technology, 89

Community service. *See also* Volunteering; as attribute for successful entry into medical school, 116

Compassion, as attribute for successful entry into medical school, 116

Competence, 17–18

Confidentiality, 41

Co-Worker Observation Reporting Systems, 185

Critical thinking, as attribute for successful entry into medical school, 115–116

Culture
of the clinic, 68–69
of medicine, xviii–xix, 1–26, 195–196
of residency, 162–164
travel and, 107
understanding differences in, 142–143
of well-being, 45

CWO. *See* Chief Wellness Officer

Cynicism, 43

DALYs. *See* Disability adjusted life years

The David Geffen School of Medicine, 116–117

Death, from suicide, xii, 109

Dementia, 79

Denial, 19

Detachment, 43

Diabetes, 58–59, 98, 106

Disability adjusted life years (DALYs), 186

Doctor–patient relationship, 89, 202

Documentation, 95–96. *See also* Electronic medical record; Time changes in, 179–180

Drug abuse, 149–167

Drummond, Mike, 208

E-consults, 59, 61, 98. *See also* Technology
technology and, 89

Education
educational interventions for implicit bias, 144
"just in time" resources in, xviii
teaching, 220–221
technology and, xviii, 17–179

Electronic medical record (EMR). *See also* "Busy work"; Documentation; Physicians
adaptation to, 199
daily messages in, 83
data included in, 176–178
demands of, xiv
improvement in use of, 73
pajama time at home and, 177–178, 204
time spent on, 35, 92, 225

Elton, Caroline, 143

Emotional depletion, 43

EMR. *See* Electronic medical record

Environment
carbon dioxide emissions in, 186–187
changes in, 186–188
climate change and health care industry, 175
physical structures and equipment, 187

Evansly, Dr., 112–113

Facebook, 108

Family, of physicians, 5–6, 36

Federation of Medical Boards, 48–49

Fidelity, 18

Galvin, Brett, 194–214

Galvin, Cathy, 194–214

Garcia, Dr., 78

Garcia, Luis, 101–124

Generation X, 24

Google, 231

Gordon, Brian, 28

Hall, David, 116

Haney, Susan, 47

HappyMD, 208
Harrod, Dr., 125–139
Harvard University, xv
Hawley, Nigel, 226
Health care industry, xv–xviii
  business model for, 220
  changes in, 186–188
  "change toxicity" of, 65
  climate change and, 175
  communication, 33
  costs of, xv, 97–98
  efficiency of, 34
  finances of, 74, 167
  leadership in, 19–20
  LGBT individuals and, 131
  medically driven leadership in, xvii
  mission statement of, 57, 66
  proposed changes in, 34
  proposed organizational strategies in, 45
  Quadruple Aim, 43–44
  social justice in, 21
  strategic planning in, 72
  success of, 66
  Triple Aim, 43–44
  workflow improvements in, 69, 70
Health Professionals Advancing LGBTQ Equality (Gay and Lesbian Medical Association), 141
Heroin, addiction to, 153
Hippocratic Oath, xix, 16–17
  proposed changes to, 17–18
Holistic review, 117
Hope, 17
Hospital care, 187
Howard, Mr., 101–124
Huddle Implementation, 63–64, 68

IDP. *See* Independent development plan
IEDs. *See* Improvised explosive devices
IHI. *See* Institute for Healthcare Improvement

Implicit bias
  consequences of, 142
  description of, 140–146
  educational interventions for, 144
  IHI strategies to reduce, 142
  solutions to the problem of, 142
  teaching about, 143
Improvised explosive devices (IEDs), 134
Independent development plan (IDP), 83–84
  long-term goals of, 84–85
Innovation, case vignette on, 77–99
Institute for Healthcare Improvement (IHI), 43
  strategies to reduce implicit bias, 142
Intellectualization, 19
Isla, Lindy, 55, 58, 67, 77–99

Jackson, Ellen, 215–233
Jameston, Bill, 28
Johns Hopkins, xv
The Joint Commission, 28, 142
"Joy of Medicine" program, 231–232
Justice, 18
  social, 21

Kaiser Family Foundation, 23
Kaiser Permanente, xv
Kirch, Darrell, xvi–xviii, 123
Krebs cycle, 113

Lawsuits
  long-term impact on physicians, 23
  against physicians, 7–8, 22–23
Leadership
  as attribute for successful entry into medical school, 117
  description of, 72
  programs for, 71–72
Leadership in Energy and Environmental Design (LEED)-certified buildings, 187

Lean Six Sigma Accreditation, 63
LEED. *See* Leadership in Energy and
    Environmental Design-certified
    buildings
Legislation
    Affordable Care Act, xvi
    Americans with Disabilities Act,
        48–49
    Paris Accord, 187
LGBT individuals
    health care and, 131
    in medical school, 132–139
Life span, of physicians, x–xi
Lifestyle
    changes in, 152, 205
    of physician, 24
Losara, Dr., 129

Malpractice Reports, 22
Management
    description, 72
    physician involvement in
        decisions, 73
Marijuana, 153
Marriage
    medical, 193–214
    successful, 217
Mayo Clinic, xv, 43
MCAT, 107
Medical Board of California, 230
    licensing requirements, 47–49
Medical license. *See* U.S. Medical
    Licensing Exam
Medical marriage, xx
    case vignette of, 193–214
    finances during, 211–212
    negative side of, 210
    principles of, 209–211
Medical school
    admission teams, 115
    attributes for successful entry into,
        115–116
    changes in admission process,
        144–145
    core competencies for prepared-
        ness for, **117**

    joy and meaning in, 225–226
    multiple mini-interview format,
        144–145
    preprofessional competencies as
        attribute for successful entry
        into medical school, 117
    process of admission, 102–124
    surviving, 120
    teaching about implicit bias in, 143
    unbiased advice to students, 117
    well-being curriculum and biases
        in, 125–146
Medical students
    debt relief program for, 81
    influence of mentors on, 130–131
    mental health of, xii
    suicide and, 132
    support system and, 113
Medicine
    alternative careers in, 185–186
    culture of, xviii–xix, 1–26, 195–196
    defining meaning in, 169–190
    joy and meaning of, 215–234
    medical marriages, 193–214
    medical societies, 230–233
    "old style," 55
    physician transition to retirement
        from, 218–219
    podcasts, 217–218, 224
    pre-med vulnerability and
        trauma, 101–124
    unintended consequences of
        culture of, 18–19
    virtual, 169–190
Medscape, 22
Mental health
    of medical students, xii
    of physicians, xii, 37
    stigma about, 42, 49–50
    "Triple Aim," 30
Mentees, tips for, **94**
Mentoring
    barriers to, 63
    career development plans and, 70
    case vignette on, 77–99

Mentoring *(continued)*
  implicit biases and, 95
  process of, 92
  program for, 61–62, 69
  success of, 92
Mentors
  influence on medical students,
    130–131
  residents and, 126–127
  tips for, **93**
Military, 132–133
Millennials, 24
  description of, 167
  as future physicians, 119
Mission statement, 57, 66
MMI. *See* Multiple mini-interview
    format
Models. *See also* "Project Echo"
  business, 220
  financial model, 177
  physicians as role models, 76
  WellMD "professional fulfillment
    model," 45
Morale
  case vignette on, 53–76
  improvement of, 70
Morphine, 154
Multiple mini-interview (MMI)
    format, 144–145

National Academy of Medicine, 19
National Institutes of Health,
    xvii–xviii
National Medical Association, 83
Newton, Louise, 215–233
Nonmaleficence, 18
"Note bloat," xiv

Odono, Ms., 30
Ohio State University College of
    Medicine, 143–144
Optimism, 17
Oxycontin, addiction to, 149–167

Pain, chronic, 149–167
"Paint Your School Pink," 141–142

"Pajama time," xiv
Parenting, 208–209
Paris Accord, 187
Parsons, Abbie, 222–223
Passion, as attribute for successful en-
    try into medical school, 118–119
Patient Advocacy Reporting System,
    185
Patients
  autonomy of, 21
  boundaries with, **97**
  care of, 58
  doctor–patient relationship,
    89, 202
  family and, 5–6
  letters to physicians from, 3–15
  physicians as, 165–167
  time with, 96–97
  virtual care technology and, 68
  welfare of, 1
Peers, 23
  physicians as role models, 76
Personal achievement, 43
Physicians. *See also* Electronic medi-
    cal record; Well-being
  abuse of prescribed drugs, xii
  alcohol abuse disorder in, xii
  burnout, xv, 42
  "busy work" done by, xiv
  career development plans of, 70
  case vignette on the culture of
    medicine and, 1–26
  "change laggards," 65
  "compulsive triad" of personality,
    xviii–xix
  dedication of, 2–3
  development of clinical expertise,
    98
  doctor–patient relationship, 89,
    202
  empathy from, 219
  flexibility of hours, 97
  fulfillment in career, 188–189
  "hybrid," 96
  involvement in management
    decisions, 73

"laggards," 70–71
lawsuits against, 7–8, 22–23
licensing, 74–75, 223–224
life span of, xi–xiii
lifestyle of, 24
mental health of, xii, 37
as money managers, 221–222
as patients, 165–167, 193–214
pressure on, 32
pro bono work, 230
relationships, 208
role identification of, 74
as role models, 76
schizophrenia in, xii
self-care of, 163
"street credibility" of, 56
stress and, 6–7, 180–181
transition to retirement from
    clinical practice, 218–219
volunteering during retirement,
    219, 230–231
"walk the talk" of, 57
Podcasts, 217–218, 224, 232
Posttraumatic stress disorder (PTSD),
    134–136
Pre-medicine, case vignette of,
    101–124
Prescription drugs, 187
    physician abuse of, xii
Press Ganey, 185
Primary care physician
    lack of, 23–24
Professionalism
    consequences of, xviii–xix
    monograph on, 20–21
    pressures of, 9, 11–12
"Project Echo," 86–89, 98–99
Psychiatrists
    as "physician's physician," 165
    support for medical students,
        127–128
PTSD. *See* Posttraumatic stress
    disorder

Quadruple Aim, 43

Racism, in medical school, 137, 140
Raley, Justin, 126–146
Rape, 135
Rea, Margaret, 163
Read, Dr., 226–227
Relationships, of physicians, 208
Research, as attribute for successful
    entry into medical school, 116
Residents
    addiction in, 149–168
    culture of, 162
    as mentors, 126–127
    preexisting psychological
        strengths and vulnerabilities
        in, 163
Resilience, 45. *See also* Retirement
    approaches to, 75
    as attribute for successful entry
        into medical school, 116
    case vignettes on, 53–76, 101–123
    change and, 71–72
    -enhancing activities, 75
Retirement
    median age of, 228
    transitioning into, 218–219
    volunteering during, 219, 230–231
Richmond, Paul, 1–26
Road to Resilience, 75
Roberts, Dr., 62
Royal College of Physicians and Sur-
    geons of Canada, 21

Sacramento Sierra Valley Medical
    Society, 122
Safety, 98
Schizophrenia, prevalence in
    physicians, xii
Seija, Luis E., 119
Self-care, 163
    as attribute for successful entry
        into medical school, 116
Seview, Dr., 84
Sex, in medical marriages, 198
Shaper, Jack, 53–76, 81
Sierra, Roseanne, 28–29

Sierra Sacramento Valley Medical Society (SSVMS), 228
"Silver tsunami," xvii
Six Sigma, training, 69
Sleep, deprivation, 136, 157–158
Social justice, 21
Social media, AAMC's review of social media and application to medical school, 119–120
SSVMS. See Sierra Sacramento Valley Medical Society
Stanford University, 43
Stanford Wellness Framework, 70, 92
STEM (science, technology, engineering, and mathematics), 103
"Steps Forward," 63–64
Stone, Dr., 29
Stress. See also Medical marriage
   in physicians, 6–7, 19–20, 32, 180–181
   of physicians, 6–7, 19–20, 32
   technology for prevention of, 86
Suicide, xii, 109
   in family of physician, 36
   by a medical student, 132–139
   planned, 203
   rates of, xii
   thoughts about, 165, 201

Teaching, 220–221
Teamwork, 97
Technology. See also E-consults
   education and, xviii
   to increase efficiency and reduce burnout levels, 95–96
   mobile, **97**
   "phone tag," **97**
   for prevention of burnout and stress, 86
   training and, 178–179
   use of with patients, 96, **97**
   virtual care through, 68
   well-being and, 59–60

Telemedicine, 96, 169–190
   flexibility of, 181–182
   to help physicians work differently, 184–185
   safety of, 98
Texas A&M College of Medicine, 119–120
Texas Tech University Health Sciences Center El Paso, 118
Time. See also Documentation; Electronic medical record
   after scheduled work hours, 204
   flexibility of physician hours, 97
   with patients, 96–97
Tobin, Dr., 55–56
"Triple Aim," 30
Trust, case vignette on, 77–99
Twitter, 103

UC. See University of California
UCH. See University City Health
University City Health (UCH), 27–52
University of California (UC), xv, 187
University of California, Davis, 120, 145, 163
University of California, Los Angeles, 116–117
University of Queensland, Australia, 115
U.S. Medical Licensing Exam (USMLE), 120, 133

Vanderbilt Center for Patient and Professional Advocacy, 185
Veracity, 18
Vine, Jordan, 194, 199–214
Volunteering, 219, 230–231. See also Community service
Volunteer Physician Registry, 230

Wall Street Physician, 229
Well-being
   AAMC's perspective on clinician, 145

aims of, 44
culture of, 45
curriculum in medical school,
    125–146
"curriculum" topics for, 145–146
interventions for, 189–190
lifelong learning about, xv
as motivation for career choice,
    112
overview, xiii
physician, 31
programs for, 217–218

support for, 114
technology and, 59–60
WellMD "professional fulfillment
    model," 45
Wetzel, Aileen, 231–233
Workaholics, 198
Work-life balance, 62, 67, 167, 169–190
    in medical marriage, 198
    working after hours, **97**
Workload, variety of, 96
World Health Organization, 43